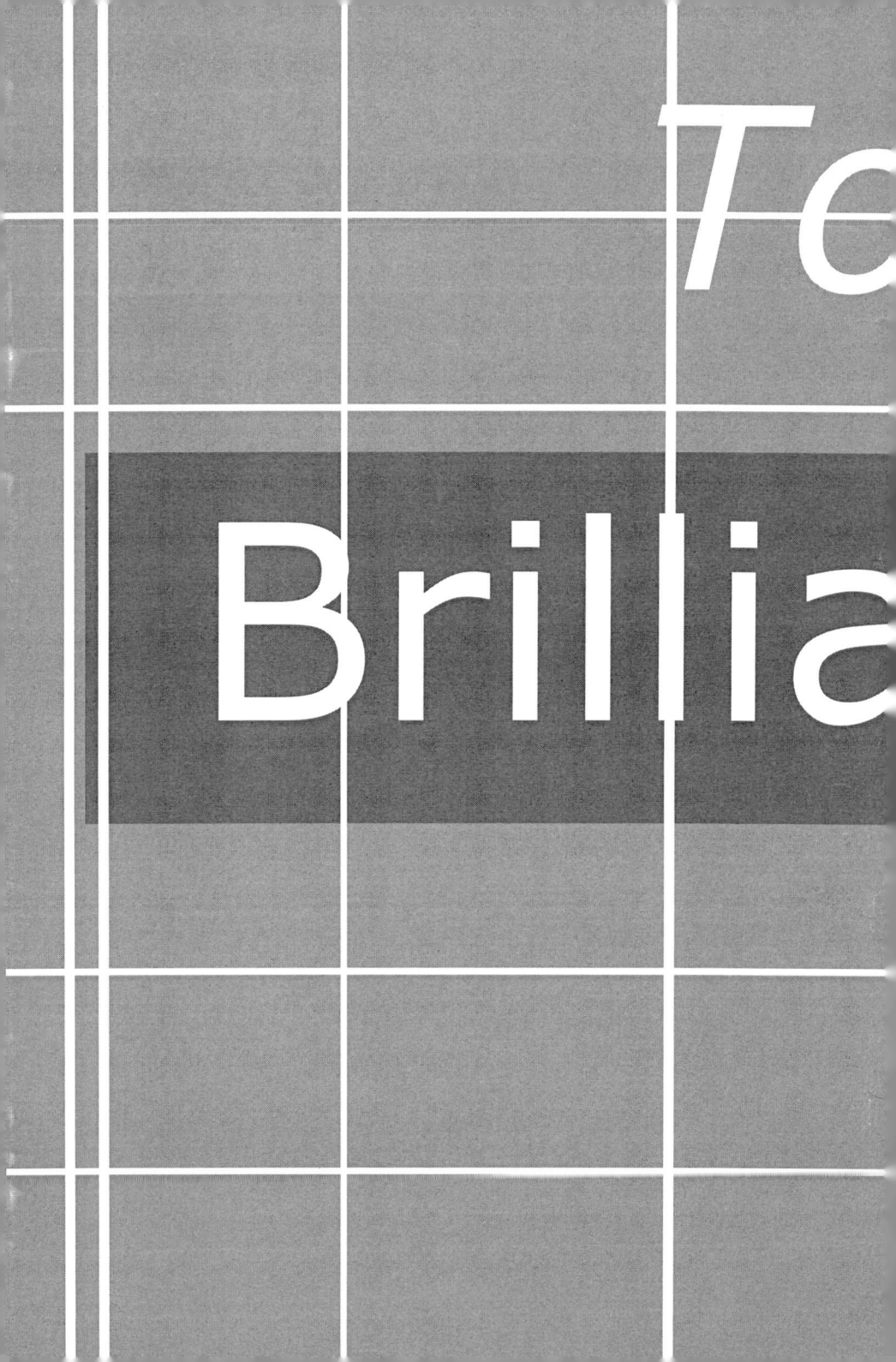

Contents

Three phases of the application process 13

Entry Examinations 13

Graduate Entry 16

Medical School entry requirements 20

Premedical Entry Programmes 31

Graduate Entry Programmes 34

Choosing a medical school 8

Making the most of your application form . . . 42

The Personal Statement 45

Examples of personal statements 51

Interview advice 74

Pre-interview Preparation 74

General advice 75

Interview structure 77

The Ethical Scenario. 77

Topical subjects likely to come up in the interview . . 80

The pre-interview video 87

One hundred and ten sample
medical school interviews 90

A collection of additional questions previously
used in interviews 167

Positive behavioural indicators 185

One hundred possible interview questions Answered . 187

Index 274

Chapter 1

Why Do You Want To be a Doctor
The Application Process
Medical Schools Entry Requirements in the UK
Premedical Entry Programmes
Graduate Entry Programmes
The UCAS Form
The Personal Statement
Sample Personal Statements

Introduction

Why do you want to be a doctor

I had an interesting afternoon recently with my group of general practice trainees. I asked them, to tell the group what their current role was in hospital medicine and why they had decided to become General Practitioners. I was slightly disappointed to discover that the vast majority said that they were looking forward to having weekends off and earning lots of money. Honest, if not heart warming!

Most applicants have a more altruistic reason for entering medicine, at least that is what they tell the interview board and I suspect most are genuine!

So why do you want to be a doctor If it is the money, you will certainly earn a reasonable living, in certain specialities you may earn a considerable living, but you will work hard for it and if money motivates you then the city may be for you.

If it is kudos that excites you, medicine is still a highly respected profession and one that scores highly in the annual 'who do you trust and respect' polls. Here politics and journalism are careers to avoid.

If it the urge to help a person that draws you, medicine can certainly fit the bill but so can nursing, policing and the cloth.

If you want a challenging occupation that pays a reasonable wage and demands a degree of problem solving and offers a huge array of different roles from dealing with the remains of the dead (pathology) to delivering the newborn (obstetrics) then perhaps we are getting warmer. One school pupil to whom I recently gave a lecture asked me if there were any areas of medicine they could enter where they did not need to speak to patients! Well, there is pathology but medicine may not be for you if you find the prospect of talking to patients a trial you would rather avoid.

Medicine is generally hard work and demands a degree of selflessness. When my son ripped open his knee recently putting the joint capsule (and his sporting career) at risk, a selfless orthopaedic surgeon cancelled his trip to the theatre (one which he had re booked after a similar event) and risked the wrath of his long suffering wife to spend the evening in theatre washing it out and repairing it.

If you spend your career in one of the branches of hospital medicine you will be expected to share in the emergency cover of the hospital, along with your colleagues, for 365 days a year, 24 hours a day, typically covering one night or weekend in every four or five as well as working in the daytime.

During your training years you will work about 50-60 hour weeks, much reduced from the 120-hour weeks worked by my peers but you will work much more intensively, covering a greater number of patients.

So why does anyone do it? Well, you will work with like minded doctors, nurses and therapists, of a similar age. You will fuse together as part of a team gaining huge satisfaction from the huge learning curve experienced after passing finals. You will laugh together, for laughter is often the way doctors cope with the difficult situations they encounter, cry together and have fantastic mess parties!

You will after several years at medical school, finally be allowed to prescribe drugs, organise investigations, put drips up, take blood, talk to patients and relatives, admit patients with acute illness and begin to feel like a real doctor

You will embark on a life's work, which is constantly moving and developing. The moment you feel you have completed your apprenticeship, passing finals, passing membership of your chosen college, becoming a consultant or G.P. partner, you realise another challenge awaits.

Would I do it all again? I know of few doctors who wish they had not entered medicine although as in any profession, they enjoy telling everyone how tough it is and how much easier it is for their juniors.

So, in conclusion, if you enter medicine for the right reasons, you will thrive on it. If you just want a well paid job with kudos, where patients are an unfortunate side effect, look elsewhere, you will never be content.

How can you make such a far-reaching decision at the age of seventeen or eighteen? It seems impossible to know for sure. I would certainly talk to your General practitioner, if you have friends who are doctors or know doctors, try to speak with them, ask them what they really enjoy about their job. See if it 'floats your boat'.

What personality types suit medicine best? I think anyone can play a role in the field of medicine, the perfectionist might be best suited to an academic research role, as the uncertainty of medicine can be hard for them to accept. The hands on practical type will love the mechano set kits used by the orthopaedic specialist. Those with fine motor skills may thrill at the almost invisible suture work of the plastic surgeon. Those who enjoy solving riddles will prefer a physician or general practice role. If microscopes or 'waking the dead' titillate you then its pathology or even forensic pathology.

The Application Process

The three phases to the application process.

Phase 1

Includes the assessment of academic standards and the aptitude testing. Like all other applications you will need to apply via the University and Colleges Admissions service (UCAS). Schools differ in their mandatory requirements and the list below illustrates these requirements and is a brief comparison of the various schools.

Entry Examinations

During 2006 the majority of medical schools introduced entrance examinations, most now require UKCAT the UK clinical aptitude test and others have a further assessment examination such at the BMAT

It is essential that you complete these examinations successfully prior to forwarding your UCAS application.

Note that the deadline for sitting UKCAT is BEFORE the UCAS application deadline. For 2008 entry registration will be open from 1 May 2007 14 September 2007. The testing window will provisionally be from 4 June 2007 10 October 2007

UKCAT is used by
University of Aberdeen; Brighton and Sussex Medical School; Cardiff University; University of Dundee; University of Durham; University of East Anglia; University of Edinburgh; University of Glasgow; Hull York Medical School; Keele University; King's College London; University of Leeds; University of Leicester (5 year and GEP); University of Manchester; University of Newcastle; University of Nottingham; University of Oxford (GEP only – 6 year course: take BMAT); Peninsula Medical School (if A-Levels are older than 2

years, you must take GAMSAT); Barts and The London; University of Sheffield; University of Southampton (5 year and GEP); University of St Andrews (Bute); St George's, University of London.

The UKCAT is held in examinations centres around the country and the date of the tests can be found on the UKCAT web site, www.UKCAT.org.uk. These aptitude tests are computerised and designed to determine your aptitude for medicine and are difficult to prepare for. There is though a test paper on the UKCAT site to give you an idea of what is expected. You may find the American SAT test papers and IQ test papers will give you some useful practice for the UKCAT.

The UKCAT in 2007 will be testing a number of modalities, namely, mental ability, problem solving ability, logical reasoning, critical thinking and information management.

The BMAT (http://www.BMAT.org.uk/prepare) is a similar examination, it is a written examination and it is designed to be difficult and most will not complete the test, do not worry, it is designed to put you under time pressure.

Note that the deadline for registering for BMAT is BEFORE the UCAS application deadline. Key dates for 2008 entry are;
Closing date for requests for special versions of question papers (e.g. Braille or enlarged) Friday, 14th September 2007
Standard entry closing date Friday, 28th September 2007
Late entry closing date (subject to penalty fees) Thursday, 11th October 2007
Test Date Wednesday, 31st October 2007
Results Release to Centres/Candidates Friday, 30th November 2007
Closing date for Results Enquiries Friday, 11th January 2008
Used by
Cambridge (6 year course and GEP); Imperial, UCL and Oxford (6 year only GEP take UKCAT).
Please note that it is not essential for applicants to the Cambridge

Graduate Course to sit the BMAT, although applicants could use a successful result as part of their premedical requirements.

The following advice comes from the BMAT website.

Section 1 tests generic skills often used in undergraduate study, including Problem Solving, Understanding Arguments and Data Analysis and Inference abilities.

Section 2 is restricted to material normally encountered in non specialist school Science and Mathematics courses (i.e. up to and including National Curriculum Key Stage 4, Double Science and Higher Mathematics).

Section 3 consists of a choice of three short essay questions of which one must be answered.
Everything that you need to prepare for the BMAT is on, or mentioned, on this web site, and you can practise the test with the specimen papers available for down load.

Section 1: Many of the multiple choice questions in this section are similar to those found in the multiple choice section of the Critical Thinking A level. If you can, get hold of some past questions or have a look at a book on Critical Thinking to help familiarise yourself with the exam and how to approach the questions.
Section 2: This tests scientific knowledge up to GCSE Double Award level however, bear in mind that it may include topics that were not in your syllabus, but in those from other exam boards, so it might be worth going through a revision guide covering several boards. Looking at past versions of this exam (such as on the BMAT website or at UCL's LAPT site, click on Exercise Menu) may help you as the questions are different from GCSE as they are designed to 'stretch' your GCSE knowledge. It is very difficult to finish this part of the exam in the time limit.
Section 3: you have half an hour to write a one page essay so make sure you take time to plan it out properly have a practice beforehand

from the past paper on the BMAT site to see how you could best divide up your time.

Remember that the BMAT is a test designed to differentiate between candidates who are academically able to begin with, so expect it to be challenging. You must ensure that you complete the correct examination for the medical school you are applying for

MSAT
Used by;
Graduate Entry Programme exam (Barts and The London, Warwick, Kings College London).
Exam format
MSAT consists of three discrete components, in multiple choice format. These are:
Critical reasoning (45 questions in 65 minutes);
Interpersonal understanding (55 questions in 55 minutes);
Written communication (2 tasks of 30 minutes each).

Graduate Entry

Increasingly people are opting to take Medicine as a second degree. This might be because they were orientated to the arts when at school or perhaps they missed the grades at A level but performed well at under graduate level and so now fulfil the academic criteria. I believe there are considerable benefits to both patients and medics in being a postgraduate. You are more mature, worldly wise and experienced. You can relate better to older patients, cope with the dramatic experiences that medicine throws up and have both worked out a successful method of learning vast quantities of information but have also moved on from the 'vomit in the gutter after the party' phase that most undergraduates go through as a right of passage.

If you wish to enter as a postgraduate you may well be asked to take the GAMSAT test as an alternative to the UKCAT or BMAT. The following advice is derived from the GAMSAT website, www.gamsat.co.uk run by Gradmed, who run courses for GAMSAT.

St George's Hospital Medical School introduced the Graduate Australian Medical School Admissions Test to the UK in 1999.
The test was initially pioneered and used in Australia 1996 by four medical schools offering graduate entry programmes. The role of GAMSAT is to assist in the selection criteria primarily for students who are applying to study medicine on the new fast track graduate entry programmes.
It is a test that draws upon wide ranging content requiring a general knowledge base that manifests a broad spectrum of skills and aptitudes. Whilst GAMSAT is predominantly multiple choice based, it places great emphasis on reasoning ability and critical thinking. It effectively gives a 360-degree overview of ability to master information adeptly and select relevant responses within a limited time frame. It actively encourages a lateral thinking approach, thinking 'outside of the box' and exploration of wider parameters in achieving solutions. After all, the study and practice of medicine demands the ability to sift through, interpret and make swift judgements from ever increasing quantities of information and data. The art of mental juggling is one that doctors perfect, and dealing with the rigours of GAMSAT is certainly an introduction to this skill.

The ability to apply conceptual thought to a broad arena of issues and reason the optimum response within pressurised time constraints is at the core of the test's requirements. A base of scientific knowledge is necessary in order to understand two things. First of all, the scenarios under question and secondly, the terminology, its meaning and application. Once a sufficient background has been acquired, then a combination of thought processes should be able to determine the most appropriate response. It isn't always black and white; in fact, it is often the reverse. But it is that ability to sort through the shades of grey with relative speed that leads to a successful outcome.

The test is divided into three sections:

Section I Reasoning in Humanities and Social Sciences

75 Questions 1 hour 40 minutes
Section II Written Communication
2 x 30 minutes essays
Section III Reasoning in Biological and Physical Sciences
110 Questions 2 hours 50 minutes
(Biology 40%, Chemistry 40% and Physics 20%)

Section
I this section comprises multiple choice questioning based on passages on a variety of topics taken from the humanities and social sciences. The section evaluates ability to think critically, comprehend and reason.
Section
II This component asks candidates to select 2 quotations from a number based on the same theme. It appraises ability to constructively draw together concepts and express ideas fluently in the written form.
Section
III This section contains multiple choice questions that are focused on passages and graphical displays or pictorial representations of data. The questions measure problem solving aptitudes with regard to scientific scenarios, to offer hypotheses, to extrapolate reasoned conclusions, and to identify connections between given variables.

Phase 2

Includes the assessment of the personal and referee' statement and the short listing for interview.

Phase 3
Is the interview process

Medical Schools Entry Requirements in the UK

Medical School entry requirements

Aberdeen
Admissions (Medicine), College Office, Polwarth Building, Foresterhill, Aberdeen, AB25 2ZD, Tel: 01224 554975
f.a.galloway@abdn.ac.uk
Entrance Exam: UKCAT
A levels: Minimum of 3 subjects. Chemistry plus at least one from Biology, Mathematics or Physics preferred (at least one from the list required). General Studies excluded. Typical Offer AAB
GCSEs: Grade A/B minimum average preferred (especially in Science subjects). Grade C minimum in English required. Maths and Biology strongly recommended. Physics (or Dual Award Science) recommended.

Barts and The London, QMUL
Undergraduate Admissions Enquiries, Barts and The London, Queen Mary's School of Medicine and Dentistry, Queen Mary, University of London, Turner Street, London E1 2AD, Tel: 020 7882 2240
medicaladmissions@qmul.ac.uk
Entrance Exam: UKCAT
A levels: Minimum of 3 subjects. Chemistry or Biology plus one further science subject required. General Studies excluded. Typical Offer AAB AS Levels: Grade B minimum in Biology or Chemistry required where not offered at full A level GCSEs: Grade B minimum in at least 6 subjects including English Language, Maths and Science

Birmingham
Admissions Tutor, Medical School, The University of Birmingham, Edgbaston, Birmingham, B15 2TT, Tel: 01214 146888 Enquiries should be through school/college C.J.Lote@bham.ac.uk
Entrance Exam: none
A levels: Minimum of 3 subjects. Chemistry and at least one from Biology, Physics or Mathematics required. General Studies excluded. Typical Offer AAB AS Levels: Grade B minimum in Biology

required GCSEs: Minimum of 8 subjects. Grade A in at least 5 subjects. Grade B minimum in English Language (or equivalent). Grade A minimum in Physics (or Dual Award Science) and Maths where not offered at A or AS Level

Brighton and Sussex
Brighton and Sussex Medical School, BSMS Teaching Building, University of Sussex, Brighton, East Sussex, BN1 9PX, Tel: 01273 644644 medadmissions@bsms.ac.uk
Entrance Exam: UKCAT
A levels: Minimum of 3 subjects. Biology or Chemistry required. General Studies excluded. Typical Offer AAB/ABB (dependant on interview performance) AS Levels: Biology (or Human Biology) and Chemistry required GCSEs: Grade B minimum in Maths & English Language (or equivalent) Base Hospital: Brighton and Sussex University Hospitals NHS Trust

Bristol
Undergraduate Admissions Office, Senate House, Tyndall Avenue, Bristol, BS8 1TH, Tel: 01179 287679 admissions@bristol.ac.uk
Entrance Exam: None
A levels: Minimum of 3 subjects. Chemistry plus one further Science required. Typical offer AAB AS Levels: For candidates offering 4 ASlevels, at least one should be in a non science subject. Typical Offer AAB GCSEs: Grade A/A passes are an advantage but there is no minimum requirement Course Information

Cambridge
University of Cambridge, University of Cambridge, Intercollegiate Admissions Office, Kellet Lodge, Tennis Court Road, Cambridge CB2 1QJ, Tel: 01223 333308 admissions@cam.ac.uk
Entrance Exam: BMAT
A levels: All colleges strongly prefer applicants to have Chemistry A level. All colleges prefer applicants to have two science/ mathematics subjects at A level note that most applicants for Medicine at Cambridge have at least 4 full A levels, with three science/

mathematics A levels. Typical Offer AAA AS Levels: Chemistry required. Pass required in a minimum of 3 from Biology, Chemistry, Physics and Maths GCSEs: Grade C minimum in Maths and Science Further Information: For individual college requirements and information consult Cambridge website

Cardiff

Admissions Officer, Medical School Office, Cardiff University, Heath Park Campus, Cardiff CF14 4XN, Tel: 029 2074 2310 medicaladmissions@cf.ac.uk
Entrance Exam: UKCAT
A levels: Minimum of 3 subjects. Grade A in Biology or Chemistry required. One further science subject or Maths must be offered. Typical offer AAB AS Levels: Grade B minimum in Biology or Chemistry required where not offered at full A level. Two AS subjects may replace a 3rd A level GCSEs: Grade AA in Dual Award Science or AAB in separate sciences required. Grade B minimum in English or Welsh Language and Maths plus at least 4 further subject

Dundee

University of Dundee, The Admissions Officer, Faculty of Medicine & Dentistry, University of Dundee, Dundee, DD1 4HN, Tel: 01382 344160 srs@dundee.ac.uk
Entrance Exam: UKCAT
A levels: Minimum of 3 subjects. Chemistry plus one further science subject required. Typical Offer AAA GCSEs: Biology (or "a good pass" in Dual Award Science) required if not offered at AS/Alevel

Durham (Stockton Campus)

Admissions Office, Durham University, Queen's Campus, University Boulevard, Stockton-on-Tees, TS17 6BH, Tel: 01913 340353 helen.taylor3@durham.ac.uk
Entrance Exam: UKCAT
A levels: Grade A minimum in at least 3 subjects, to include Biology or Chemistry at A2 or AS level. General Studies is excluded. Typical offer AAA AS Levels: Biology and Chemistry required GCSEs:

Grade C minimum in at least 5 subjects, to include English, Maths and Science (Dual Award or Separate Biology/Chemistry/Physics)

East Anglia
MB/BS Admissions Secretary, Institute of Health, Edith Cavell Building, University of East Anglia, Norwich, NR4 7TJ, Tel: 01603 591072 med.admiss@uea.ac.uk
Entrance Exam: UKCAT
A levels: Minimum of 3 subjects. Biology (or human biology) required. General studies excluded. Typical Offer AAB AS Levels: Grade B minimum in at least 1 further AS level subject GCSEs: Grade B minimum in at least 5 subjects, to include English, Maths and Science

Edinburgh
MBChB Admissions, College of Medicine and Veterinary Medicine, University of Edinburgh, The Chancellor's Building, 49 Little France Crescent, Edinburgh, EH16 4SB, Tel: 01312 426407 medug@ed.ac.uk
Entrance Exam: UKCAT
A levels: Minimum of 3 subjects. Chemistry plus at least one of Maths, Biology or Physics is required. Typical offer AAAb AS Levels: Grade B minimum. Biology is required if not offered at full A level GCSEs: Grade B minimum in Chemistry, Biology (Dual Award Science may replace sciences), Maths, English & a language other than English

Glasgow
University of Glasgow, Admissions Committee, Faculty of Medicine, University of Glasgow, Glasgow, G12 8QQ, Tel: 01413 306216 admissions@clinmed.gla.ac.uk
Entrance Exam: UKCAT
A levels: Minimum of 3 subjects. Biology and Chemistry required. General Studies excluded. Typical Offer AAB AS Levels: 4 AS level passes are expected. Preference given to applicants offering AS level English GCSEs: Grade C minimum in English. Preference given

to students offering grade A in English, Maths and Science (Dual Award or Separate Biology/Chemistry/Physics)

Hull York
Hull York Medical School Admissions, The University of Hull, Hull, HU6 7RX, Tel: 01904 321690 admissions enquiries, general enquiries
Entrance Exam: UKCAT
A levels: Minimum of 3 subjects. Biology at grade A, plus Chemistry required (except in exceptional circumstances). General Studies excluded. Typical Offer AAB AS Levels: Minimum of 4 subjects studied GCSEs: Grade C minimum in at least 6 subjects. Grade B minimum in English Language, Maths and Science (Dual Award or Separate Biology/Chemistry/Physics)

Imperial College London
Imperial College School of Medicine, The Admissions Officer, Imperial College School of Medicine, Exhibition Road, London, SW7 2AZ, Tel: 020 7594 8056 admitmed@imperial.ac.uk
Entrance Exam: BMAT
A levels: Minimum of 3 subjects. Biology or Chemistry required plus one further Science subject or Maths required. Typical Offer AABb, or AABC where 4 full A levels are offered AS Levels: Minimum of 4 subjects. Biology and Chemistry required GCSEs: 3 subjects at grade A plus 2 at grade B minimum to include English Language, Maths and Science (may be either Dual Award or Separate Biology/Chemistry/Physics)

Keele
Keele University, School of Medicine, Keele University campus, Staffordshire, ST5 5BG, Tel: 01782 583937 medicine@hfac.keele.ac.uk
Entrance Exam: UKCAT
A levels: Minimum of 3 subjects. Biology or Chemistry required plus one further Science subject or Maths required. Typical Offer: AAB AS Levels: Grade B minimum in Chemistry required if not

offered at full A level GCSEs: Grade A minimum in 4 subjects, with grade B minimum in English Language, Maths and Science (may be either Dual Award or Separate Biology/Chemistry/Physics). "A broad spread of subjects are expected at GCSE"

Kings College London
King's College London School of Medicine, First Floor, Hodgkin Building, Guy's Campus, London, SE1 1UL, Tel: 020 7848 6501
guysadmissions@kcl.ac.uk
Entrance Exam: UKCAT
A levels: Minimum of 3 subjects. Chemistry or Biology required. Typical Offer AABc AS Levels: Grade B minimum in Biology or Chemistry required if not offered at full A level GCSEs: Grade B minimum in English and Maths if not offered at A/AS level

Lancaster
Ruth Hutchison, Centre for Medical Education, Faraday Building, Lancaster University, Lancaster, LA1 4YA, Tel: 01524 594547 cme@lancaster.ac.uk UCAS Institution Code: L41 (application is via Liverpool University)
Entrance Exam: None
A levels: Minimum of 3 subjects. Biology and Chemistry required. General Studies not accepted at full A level. Typical offer AABb AS Levels: Grade B minimum required. General Studies acceptable at AS level Further Information: Applications are made through Liverpool University, applicants should indicate course code A105 to study at Lancaster. Students may apply to both Liverpool and Lancaster Base Hospital: University Hospitals of Morecambe Bay

Leeds
Admissions and Electives Office, School of Medicine, Room 7.10 Worsley Building, University of Leeds, Leeds, LS2 9JT, Tel: 01133 437194 ugmadmissions@leeds.ac.uk
Entrance Exam: UKCAT
A levels: Minimum of 3 subjects. Chemistry required. General Studies excluded. Typical Offer AAB GCSEs: Grade B minimum in

at least 6 subjects including English, Maths & Dual Award Science (or Biology and Chemistry)

Leicester
Leicester School of Medicine, Medical School Office, Maurice Shock Medical Sciences Building, University of, Leicester, PO Box 138, University Road, Leicester, LE1 9HN, Tel: 01162 522969 medadmis@le.ac.uk Entrance Exam: UKCAT
A levels: Minimum of 3 subjects. Grade A in Chemistry required. General Studies excluded. Typical Offer AAB AS Levels: Minimum of 4 subjects. Biology and Chemistry required GCSEs: Grade C minimum in English Language, Maths and Science (Dual Award or Separate Biology/Chemistry/Physics)

Liverpool
Faculty of Medicine, Faculty Support Office, The University of Liverpool, Duncan Building, Daulby St, Liverpool, L69 3GA, Tel: 0151 7064266 mbchb@liv.ac.uk
Entrance Exam: None
A levels: Minimum of 3 subjects. Biology and Chemistry required. Typical offer AABb (The A's have to be in Chemistry and Biology with the B in the 3rd subject.) AS Levels: Minimum of 4 subjects. Grade B required in AS subject not offered at full A level. General Studies acceptable at AS level. In exceptional circumstances AS grade A in Biology or Chemistry may be accepted in place of a full A level in that subject GCSEs: Grade B minimum in at least 7 subjects including English, Maths and Science (Dual Award or Separate Biology/Chemistry/Physics)

Manchester
Admissions Office, University of Manchester Medical School, Stopford Building, Oxford Road, Manchester, M13 9PT, Tel: 0161 275 5025 admissions enquiries, general enquiries UCAS Institution Code: M20
Entrance Exam: UKCAT
A levels: Minimum of 3 "rigorous" subjects (i.e. 60% minimum

theoretical content). Chemistry plus at least one from Biology (or human biology), Physics or Maths required. Typical Offer AAB GCSEs: Minimum of 7 passes. Grade A required in at least 4 subjects. Grade B minimum in English Language required. Grade C minimum in Biology, Chemistry, Physics (or grade BB in Dual Award Science) and Maths required Base Hospitals: Central Manchester & Manchester Children's University Hospitals NHS Trust (MRI), Salford Royal Hospitals NHS Foundation Trust (Hope), South Manchester University Hospitals NHS Trust (Wythenshawe), Lancashire Teaching Hospitals NHS Foundation Trust (Preston) Further Information: Predominantly PBL course. Students do cadaveric wholebody dissection anatomy teaching in years 1 & 2. Early Experience clinical contact from year 1

Newcastle Upon Tyne
University of Newcastle, The Administrative Assistant (Admissions), Medical School Framlington Place, University of Newcastle Upon Tyne, Newcastle Upon Tyne, NE2 4HH, Tel: 0191 222 7034 enquiries@ncl.ac.uk Entrance Exam: UKCAT
AS/Alevels: Biology or Chemistry required at AS or A level. Applicants are required to achieve 30 points minimum (where A level grade A=10, B=8, C=6, etc. AS grades score half points). General Studies and Critical Thinking excluded. Typical offer AAA GCSEs: Grade C minimum in at least 5 subjects. Where Biology or Chemistry is not offered at AS/Alevel grade A minimum is required in that subject (or Dual Award Science)

Nottingham
Medical School Faculty Office, The University of Nottingham, Queen's Medical Centre, Nottingham, NG7 2UH, Tel: 0115 823 0000 medschool@nottingham.ac.uk
Entrance Exam: UKCAT
A levels: Minimum of 3 subjects. Grade A minimum in Biology and Chemistry. General Studies excluded. Typical Offer AAB AS Levels: Grade A minimum in Biology and Chemistry GCSEs: Grade A minimum in at least 6 subjects including Chemistry, Biology and

Physics (or Dual Award Science). Grade A at AS Level Physics can compensate for achieving grade B at GCSE. Grade B minimum in Maths and English Language required

Oxford
University of Oxford, The Coordinator for Admissions, University of Oxford Medical School, Oxford, OX1 3RE, Tel: 01865 285783 admissions enquiries, general enquiries
Entrance Exam: BMAT
A levels: Minimum of 3 subjects. Chemistry plus at least one of Biology, Physics or Maths required. Typical Offer AAA GCSEs: Grade C minimum in Biology, Physics and Maths where not offered at A level

Peninsula
The Peninsula Medical School, The John Bull Building, Tamar Science Park, Research Way, Plymouth, PL6 8BU, Tel: 01752 437444 pmsenq@pms.ac.uk
Entrance Exam: UKCAT
AS/Alevels: Offer based on a maximum of 4 AS/Alevel subjects. Grade A required in at least one science subject. General Studies excluded. Typical offer 370400 UCAS tariff points (320 points minimum from 3 full A levels) AS Levels: Grade C minimum in at least 4 subjects GCSEs: Grade C minimum in at least 7 subjects including English Language and Maths Base Hospital Locations: Exeter, Plymouth and Truro

Queens University Belfast
Doctor D.R. McCluskey, School of Medicine Admissions, Queen's University Belfast, 73 University Road, Belfast, Northern Ireland, BT7 1NN, Tel: 028 9063 2707 s.clinmed@qub.ac.uk
Entrance Exam: None
A levels: Minimum of 3 subjects. Chemistry plus at least one of Biology, Physics or Maths required. General Studies excluded. Typical Offer AAAa AS Levels: Grade A minimum. Biology is required where not offered at full A level. GCSEs: Grade C

minimum in English Language required. Maths and Physics (or Dual Award Science) required where not offered at AS/Alevel. Performance in best 9 GCSEs is considered when assessing applicants. Candidates should offer at least 4 A grades. A poor performance at GCSE may be compensated for by strong AS/Alevel performance.

Sheffield

Doctor M S Lennard, Undergraduate Dean for Medical Admissions, School of Medicine and Biomedical Sciences, University of Sheffield, Beech Hill Road, Sheffield, S10 2RX, Tel: 0114 271 3727 medadmissions@sheffield.ac.uk
Entrance Exam: UKCAT
A levels: Chemistry plus one further Science required. Typical Offer AAB (or AAA for resit candidates) AS Levels: Grade ABBB minimum in 4 subjects. Biology and Chemistry plus one of Maths or Physics required. GCSEs: Grade A minimum in at least 4 subjects. Grade C minimum in English, Maths and Science (Dual Award or Separate Biology/Chemistry/Physics)

Southampton

Medical Admissions Office, Biomedical Sciences Building, University of Southampton, Bassett Crescent East, Southampton, SO16 7PX, Tel: 02380 594408 bmadmissions@soton.ac.uk
Entrance Exam: UKCAT
AS/Alevels: Grade B minimum in Chemistry at full A level OR grade B minimum in Biology and Chemistry at AS level required. General Studies excluded. Subjects where there may be considerable overlap of material will not be accepted in combination (such as combinations of Zoology, Biology or Physical Education; Maths, Further Maths, or Pure Maths). Typical offer AAB GCSEs: Grade B minimum in at least 7 subjects including English, Maths and Science

St. Andrews (Bute)

Medical Admissions Officer, University of St Andrews Admissions Application Centre, St Katherine's West, The Scores, St Andrews, Fife, KY16 9AX, Tel: 01334 462150 admissions@standrews.ac.uk

Entrance Exam: UKCAT
A levels: Chemistry plus at least one of Biology, Physics or Maths required GCSEs: Grade B minimum in English, Maths and Biology required where not offered at AS/Alevel (Dual Award Science is not acceptable where GCSE Biology is required) Further Information: Students undergo a 3-year Bachelor of Science(Hons) Medicine degree at St Andrews, after which they undergo clinical training usually in conjunction with Manchester University Medical School or another Scottish Medical School

St George's
Admissions Office, St George's Hospital Medical School, Cranmer Terrace, London, SW17 0RE, Tel: 020 8672 9944 medicine@sgul.ac.uk
Entrance Exam: UKCAT
A levels: Minimum of 3 subjects. Biology or Chemistry required. General Studies excluded. Typical offer AABb (this may be lowered in certain circumstances) AS Levels: Minimum of 4 subjects. Biology or Chemistry required where not offered at full A level GCSEs: Minimum of 8 subjects including Maths, English and Science scoring an average of grade A. Grade B in English Language (or IELTS 7.0) required

University College London
Undergraduate Admissions Tutor, The Royal Free and University College Medical School, Gower Street, London, WC1E 6BT, Tel: 020 7679 0841 medicaladmissions@ucl.ac.uk
Entrance Exam: BMAT
A levels: Minimum of 3 subjects. Chemistry required. "Some preference will be given to applicants who, in addition to Chemistry and Biology, offer a contrasting subject at A or ASlevel". Typical Offer AAB AS Levels: Minimum of 4 subjects. Biology required where not offered at full A level. General Studies acceptable at AS level only GCSEs: Grade B minimum in English Language and Maths required Base Hospital: Royal Free Hampstead NHS Trust Further Information: Resit candidates are not considered

Premedical Entry Programmes

Premedical Entry Programmes comprise of the standard 5 year medical course, with an extra 'Foundation year' at the start of the course (bringing the total length of the course to 6 years, not including any time spent intercalating).

Typical premedical entry students are those who have taken non science A levels, or qualifications which are not considered for entry to standard 5 year programs. Graduates may also apply to these programs, particularly if their degree has little or no scientific content. Students who have taken Chemistry at A level are generally not allowed to apply for premedical courses, although some universities allow those with a Biology A level to apply.

The foundation year of the course serves to prepare students for entry into a typical medical degree. Programmes may comprise of Chemistry, Biology, Physics, Maths and other subjects, with topics sometimes being related to medicine. In some medical schools a small degree of clinical experience is gained in the foundation year. Successful completion of the foundation year leads to automatic entry to the medical school's standard 5-year program. Competition for places on these courses is very severe, sometimes harder than typical 5-year courses.

The following medical schools offer Premedical courses :

Bristol
Undergraduate Admissions Office, Senate House, Tyndal Avenue, Bristol, BS8 1TH, Tel: 01179 287679 admissions@bristol.ac.uk
UCAS Course Code: A104
Entrance Exam: None Places: 10
A levels: AAB, or a 2.1 degree. No more than one science. General studies not accepted. AS Levels: Minimum of four subjects. GCSEs: Grade A/A passes are an advantage but there is no minimum requirement

Cardiff

Admissions Officer, Medical School Office, Cardiff University, Heath Park Campus, Cardiff CF14 4XN, Tel: 029 2074 2310 medicaladmissions@cf.ac.uk UCAS Course Code: A104
Entrance Exam: UKCAT Places: 16
A levels: AAB required including no more than one science subject. General Studies not accepted. AS Levels: Two AS subjects may replace a 3rd A level GCSEs: Grade AA in Dual Award Science or AAB in separate sciences required. Grade B minimum in English or Welsh Language and Maths plus at least 4 further subjects

Dundee
University of Dundee, The Admissions Officer, Faculty of Medicine & Dentistry, University of Dundee, Dundee, DD1 4HN, Tel: 01382 344160 srs@dundee.ac.uk UCAS Course Code: A104
Entrance Exam: UKCAT
A levels: AAA required, including not more than one science, or an upper second class Honours degree in a non science discipline. GCSEs: Biology (or "a good pass" in Dual Award Science) required.

Edinburgh
MBChB Admissions, College of Medicine and Veterinary Medicine, University of Edinburgh, The Chancellor's Building, 49 Little France Crescent, Edinburgh, EH16 4SB, Tel: 01312 426407 medug@ed.ac.uk UCAS Course Code: A104
Entrance Exam: UKCAT
A levels: AAA required. Only one of Maths and Further Maths will be considered. AS Levels: Grade B minimum. GCSEs: Grade B minimum in Chemistry, Maths, English & a language other than English. Double Award Combined Sciences at grade BB may replace GCSE grades in sciences. Further Information: Resit applicants not accepted (except under very extenuating circumstances)(Excludes AS level resits).

Keele
Keele University, School of Medicine, Keele University campus, Staffordshire, ST5 5BG, Tel: 01782 583937 medicine@hfac.keele.

ac.uk UCAS Course Code: B900
Entrance Exam: UKCAT A levels: AAB (Chemistry and Biology not accepted). General Studies not accepted. AS Levels: Grade B minimum in Chemistry required if not offered at full A level GCSEs: Grade C in English and Maths. Grade A minimum in 4 subjects. "A broad spread of subjects are expected at GCSE"

Kings College London
King's College London School of Medicine, First Floor, Hodgkin Building, Guy's Campus, London, SE1 1UL, Tel: 020 7848 6501 guysadmissions@kcl.ac.uk Course Length: 6 years UCAS Course Code: A103
Entrance Exam: UKCAT Places: 30 (plus 18 on Dental foundation course)
Entry Requirements: AAB/C at A/AS level. Candidates offering Chemistry at A/AS level but not Biology are not eligible, whilst candidates offering Biology but not Chemistry are. Graduates should have an upper second honours degree (or lower second if combined with a masters). Normal A/AS level requirements do not apply to graduates (i.e. AAB at A level is not required at first attempt). Applicants with other qualifications should contact the medical school.

Manchester
Admissions Office, University of Manchester Medical School, Stopford Building, Oxford Road, Manchester, M13 9PT, Tel: 0161 275 5025 admissions enquiries, general enquiries UCAS Course Code: A104
Entrance Exam: UKCAT
A levels: Grades AAB required. Two AS levels are not accepted in the place of an A level. General Studies is not accepted. GCSEs: Minimum of 7 passes. Grade A required in at least 4 subjects. Sciences required at Grade B. 'BB' in Dual Science Award acceptable. English Language required at Grade B, and Maths is essential.

Sheffield
Doctor M S Lennard, Undergraduate Dean for Medical Admissions, School of Medicine and Biomedical Sciences, University of Sheffield, Beech Hill Road, Sheffield, S10 2RX, Tel: 0114 271 3727 medadmissions@sheffield.ac.uk UCAS Course Code: A104
Entrance Exam: UKCAT
A levels: AAB (or better) in arts subjects, or a degree. General Studies 'normally acceptable'. AS Levels: Grade ABBB minimum in 4 subjects. GCSEs: GCSE Chemistry and Maths, and preferably Biology and Physics, plus higher level qualifications (i.e. non science A levels).

Graduate Entry Programmes

Graduate Entry Programmes are abridged courses (typically 4 years in duration) for people who have already done an undergraduate degree. Some schools specify your first degree should be in a science or health care related subject, while others will entertain applications from graduates of any discipline.
Competition for places is tough, however all medical schools, except SGUL and Nottingham, welcome applications to their standard and foundation courses from graduate students.

GEPs are currently offered by the following medical schools:

Barts and The London, QMUL
Graduate Entrants Programme, Student Office, Queen Mary's School of Medicine and Dentistry, Barts & The London, Old Medical College Building, Turner Street, London, E1 2AD, Tel: 020 7882 2244 gepmedicine@qmul.ac.uk Course Length: 4 years
Entrance Exam: MSAT
Entry Requirements: First or Upper Second degree in a science or a health related subject. This will usually be a Bachelor's degree, but may be a Master's, if it is a first degree Course Information

Birmingham
University of Birmingham, The Assistant Registrar, The Medical School, University of Birmingham, Birmingham B15 2TJ, Tel: 0121 414 6888 Course Length: 4 years Places: 40
Entry Requirements: First or Upper Second Class Honours degree in a life science discipline (due to high demand, for both 2003 and 2004 only candidates with first class degrees were considered). Chemistry grade C minimum at A level (or equivalent) OR Chemistry content in degree offered Further Information: Students undertake a 2 year clinical orientation course, after which they join the final 2 years of the 5-year course

Bristol
University of Bristol Admissions Office, Senate House, Tyndall Avenue, Bristol, BS8 1TH, Tel: 0117 928 7679 Course Length: 4 Years Further Information: Students follow the same premedical teaching schedule as those on the 5-year course, with the exception of the "Molecular and Cellular Basis of Medicine" unit and the year 2 SSC (certain students may also be exempt from the anatomy component). The teaching is also condensed into 1 year as opposed to the 2 year course for undergraduates. The remaining 3 (clinical) years are identical to the 5-year course

Cambridge
Cambridge Admissions Office, Fitzwilliam House, 32 Trumpington St, Cambridge, CB2 1QY, Tel: 01223 333308 Hughs Hall admissions, Lucy Cavendish College admissions, Wolfson College Admissions Course Length: 4 years Places: 20
Entrance Exam: BMAT (some applicants may be exempt)
Entry Requirements: First or Upper Second Class degree in any subject. AS/Alevel passes in Chemistry plus two from Biology, Physics and Maths. GCSE grade C minimum in Maths and Science Further Information: Open to UK and EU residents only

Kings College London

King's College London School of Medicine, First Floor, Hodgkin Building, Guy's Campus, London, SE1 1UL, Tel: 020 7848 6501 guysadmissions@kcl.ac.uk Course Length: 4 years
Entrance Exam: MSAT
Entry Requirements: First or Upper Second Class Honours degree in any subject OR Lower Second Class Honours degree with postgraduate degree in any subject OR Diploma of Higher Education in Nursing pass with at least two years nursing work experience Further Information: Suitably qualified graduate applicants applying to the four year Graduate Entry Programme who sit MSAT will also be automatically considered for the five year programme

Leicester
Doctor W Montague, Graduate Admissions Tutor, Leicester School of Medicine, Medical School Office, Maurice Shock Medical Sciences Building, University of Leicester, PO Box 138, University Road, Leicester, LE1 9HN, Tel: 0116 252 2969 medadmis@le.ac.uk

Liverpool
MBChB Admissions Office, Faculty of Medicine, Duncan Building, Daulby Street, Liverpool, L69 3GA, Tel: 0151 706 4266 mbchb@liv.ac.uk

Newcastle
Medical Student Office, Medical School, University of Newcastle upon Tyne, Newcastle upon Tyne, NE2 4HH, Tel: 0191 222 5594 enquiries@ncl.ac.uk Course Length: 4 years
Entrance Exam: UKCAT
Entry Requirements: First or Upper Second Class degree OR be a practising health professional with a post registration qualification. All applicants will be expected to provide evidence of academic endeavour within the last three years (e.g. A level study, Open University, GAMSAT) Further Information: Phase I of the programme lasts 45 weeks and provides an equivalent level of experience to the 2 pre-clinical years of the 5-year course. Phase II

(clinical) is identical to the 5-year course

Nottingham
The University of Nottingham Medical School at Derby, Derby City General Hospital, Uttoxeter Road, Derby, DE22 3DT, Tel: 01332 724622 GEM@nottingham.ac.uk
Entrance Exam: GAMSAT
Entry Requirements: Lower Second Class Honours degree minimum
Further Information: Students do an 18 month foundation course. Following completion of the foundation course students undergo a 17 week clinical practice course. This is followed by a final 2 years of clinical study

Oxford
Mrs Lesley Maitland, Medical School Office, John Radcliffe Hospital, Oxford, OX3 9DU, Tel: 01865 228975 lesley.maitland@medsci.ox.ac.uk Entrance Exam: UKCAT
Entry Requirements: Ideally a First or Upper Second Class Honours degree in any applied or experimental science. A level Chemistry plus one other science, and GCSE Biology also required unless substantially covered in degree course offered Further Information: Graduate applicants are free to apply to both Oxford and Cambridge simultaneously

Southampton
Medical Admissions Office, Biomedical Sciences Building, University of Southampton, Bassett Crescent East, Southampton, SO16 7PX, Tel: 02380 594408 bmadmissions@soton.ac.uk Course Length: 4 years
Entry Requirements: First or Upper Second Class Honours degree in any subject. A level pass in Chemistry and AS level pass in Biology (or equivalents). GCSE grade C minimum in English, Maths and Science (or equivalents) Further Information: For the first 2 years of the course, students will share some components with students on the 5-year course. In years 3 and 4 students will work alongside students from the 5-year course during clinical attachments

St George's
Michilla Regan, MBBS Admissions Officer, St George's, University of London, Cranmer Terrace, London, SW17 0RE, Tel: 020 8725 5201 gep@sgul.ac.uk Course Length: 4 years Places: 70
Entrance Exam: GAMSAT
Entry Requirements: First or Second Class Honours degree in any discipline or an MSc, MPhil or PhD. Minimum score of 62 in GAMSAT

University of Wales, Swansea
School of Medicine, Swansea University, Singleton Park, Swansea, SA2 8PP, Tel: 01792 513400 Course Length: 4 years Further Information: In Years 1 & 2 you will study an equivalent programme of study to the first three years of the 5-year course at Cardiff, and this will be over two extended academic years.

Warwick
University of Warwick, Medicine Graduate Entry Programme, Postgraduate Admissions Office, Coventry, CV4 7AL, Tel: 024 7652 4585

Choosing a medical school

Sage advice from a Manchester student, these problems are not peculiar to Manchester by any means and are designed to provide an example rather than a criticism of Manchester. The sub specialisation in subjects has led to a need to travel further to obtain training...

'Make sure you apply to a medical school because you want to go there and like the course, don't apply to the ones you simply think you're most likely to get an offer from. This is a mistake I made and looking back my choices would have been much different.
When considering where to apply, make sure you check out about clinical placements, in my case I was sent to a different city 40 miles away from Manchester for the entire duration of my clinical

training. Had I known this when I applied, I might not have applied to Manchester There are a large number of reasons for choosing a particular school;'

Further advice.
Competition for places, some schools are more popular than others but beware. Schools publish the number of applicants and what tends to happen is next years applicants all head for the least popular one making it..well, the most popular one.
Obviously location is important, proximity to home, friends and family may be very important to you, although you will find as you make friends the school life takes over from home life.
Expense can be an important factor, London is more expensive than virtually anywhere to rent and live.
Future location. One tends to find that you tend to settle around the area that you train, particularly after you leave medical school so if you have a choice of schools, take this into account.
Do you wish to live in a city or in the country? There are not many medical schools in the country but smaller cities like Bristol and Leeds are very close to surrounding country.
What are the transport links like? If you are a talented sports man and need to get to training, you will want to know it is not a three hour round trip to the site of your sport.
How does it fit in with your particular extracurricular interests. What facilities does the school or area have? Sports facilities, Cinema, Theatre, Ice Rinks / Swimming Pools
What accommodation is offered, are there halls of residence and if so for how many years. Halls are usually provided for 1st year after which you may be asked to move out to other rented accommodation. Look at cost of accommodation
What is the course structure and teaching Styles, is it problem based learning or traditional
Do they accept or encourage graduates and mature students. Are graduate degree courses offered, is an intercalated degree mandatory? How much time is spent in the community or in other hospitals? Are electives offered if so for how long and at what stage.

Is any help offered in the form of bursaries or scholarships

How frequently are examinations or assessments performed
What is the balance between theory and practice
Does it have a strong academic reputation. Purely academic doctors are NOT the best. Consider the syllabus rather than reputation, you may need to work harder at some places

What are the advantages and disadvantages of a university over a medical school?

University
Usually has a large campus, diversity of population, possibly more opportunities to go to different hospitals?
You will mix with students doing other degrees

Medical school
Is a smaller, more close knit community but has students who are all sitting the same degree

The UCAS form

Making the most of your application form

A glance at the UCAS form, will reveal that you have to give the following information:
Your personal details (name, address, nationality, how you will be funded, etc.)
Those courses and institutions you want to apply to
The qualifications you already have taken (such as GCSEs, AS-levels if certificated (see below) or equivalents)
The qualifications you will take before you enter university/college (general and vocational A-levels, BTEC, other AS-levels etc.)
And you will need to complete the personal statement.

For those courses where interviews are held, the UCAS form is used to draw up a short-list of candidates. The form is crucial in gaining you an interview.

Personal details
Write your surname in the surname/family name part, and your first name in the first/given name section.
Your date of birth is the date you were born on. It is not the date on which you filled in the form. Do not fall into the trap of filling in the date you completed the form it does not impress!

Selecting your courses and institutions

Check you have noted the correct course code for each institution, and the correct institution code.
Make sure you use the right institution code as these can be easily mistaken.
If you are dyslexic make sure that someone checks your form. Electronic and on-line applications have an automatic checking system that detects such errors.
Check that you have checked the admissions requirements for that course at that university/college, including any GCSE requirements.

For medicine (and dentistry and veterinary science), you can only apply for a maximum of 4 medical courses you are encouraged to include two non-medical courses on your form (it is recommended that these are medicine- or science-related).

Completing sections 7A and 7B

These should be listed in qualifications completed (Section 7A) and must include the following (with the dates on which the examinations were taken and the grades obtained):
1. GCSEs
2. AS-levels which have been completed and for which you have accepted certification.
3. Vocational Certificate of Education AS- or A-level which have been completed and for which you have accepted certification.
4. Any other qualifications that are relevant to the courses you are applying for.
Note: you must enter any AS- or A-levels for which you have accepted certification, even if you will carry these subjects to a full A-level or Vocational Double Award.

The qualifications you will take in the next year
These are to be entered in qualifications not yet completed (section 7B).

You should put in this section:
1. The A-levels which you are taking regardless of whether the relevant AS-level has been certificated (and listed in section 7A) or not.
2. If you are taking a full A-level, but wish to claim separate certification for the full AS-level, you should list both of these awards.
3. Any Vocational Double Awards, regardless of whether the Single Award has been certificated and is shown in section 7A.
4. Any stand-alone AS-levels which you are taking in Year 13.

5. Any stand-alone AS-levels which you started in Year 12 and will complete in Year 13 (even if you will re-take units).

7. If you are retaking all your units in an AS-level and will accept certification at the end of Year 13 (even if these units will also count towards an A-level) you should list all the AS-level units in section 7B. If you do not want separate AS-level certification then do not list these units.

8. If you are taking Advanced Extension Awards you should list these in section 7B. If you have not accepted certification for AS-levels you have taken in Year 12, then you do not list these in section 7A. If these units are to count towards a full A-level then you also do not list them separately in section 7B unless you wish to accept separate certification for these units.

How to complete sections 7A and 7B

Example 1
In Year 12, Bob the Builder took AS-levels in Maths, Chemistry, Biology and Physics. He accepted the AS-level certificates for all of these subjects and is continuing Maths, Chemistry and Biology to A-level, plus taking General Studies A-level. He fills in his UCAS form as follows:

Section 7A : GCSE results plus Examination(s)/Award(s)

Month	Year	Awarding Body	Subject	Level	Result
06	07	OCR	Maths	AS	A
06	07	OCR	Chemistry	AS	B
06	07	OCR	Biology	AS	A
06	07	OCR	Physics	AS	A

Section 7B

Month	Year	Awarding Body	Subject	Level	Result
06	08	OCR	Maths	A	
06	08	OCR	Chemistry	A	
06	08	OCR	Biology	A	
06	08	OCR	General Studies	A	

Requirements vary but at GCSE level you should have 6 grade A or better and at least a B in Maths and English and As in the three sciences. At A level most will require AAB and chemistry as a subject, Biology is preferred but not essential.

In addition to academic achievements, other qualifications may be very helpful to your application. Music, language, business skills, Young enterprise and computer skills may all help..

The Personal Statement

The following few paragraphs come from the University of Southampton website and nicely sum up what to avoid;

What to avoid

Pretentiousness: attempting to impress, you may end up out of your league ('I was totally absorbed by The Naked Ape'). Keep your style clear and simple.

Facetiousness: a touch of doctory wit can be engaging, but it's easy to hit the wrong note and cause irritation rather than amusement.

Frantic self advertisement: Don't let your positive selfpresentation tip over into immodesty ('My achievements at school were vast'; or even, 'It is my mature, collected approach to life that sets me apart from others. Due to my experiences, I tackle the tasks presented to me with wisdom and sincerity...').

We are really turned off by shaky written English: selectors are likely to take poor spelling as evidence of carelessness, and poor sentence construction as an indication of both problems with communication and a lack of feeling for style. A badly written personal statement can make the difference between acceptance and rejection, even if your reference and predictions are good.

Illegibility: write clearly, or use a 12-point font if you are word processing; bare in mind that the forms are reproduced in a reduced format for admissions tutors.

Conformity: too many personal statements are formulaic, saying what applicants feel they ought to say in a vocabulary that they feel they ought to use . Although taking advice is sensible, bear in mind the disarmingly off message comment of one of our applicants: 'Are these as tedious to read as they are to write? I'm sorry, I really feel that it is impossible to call these personal statements considering the amount of instruction we are given in writing them. We're told what to say and how to say it in an all too explicit manner." Be yourself; it's a pleasure (though a surprisingly rare one) to read a statement where the candidate's own voice comes over clearly.

What are the Admission Teams looking for?

Your suitability to take that degree course
Your motivation to study medicine
Your knowledge of the subject you are applying for.
Your other skills and experience
Admissions Tutors will look at different sections of your form to make their decisions. Obviously your current qualifications and the

ones you will take are important, and the reference from your school or college will support your academic background and your suitability for that course.

Writing a personal statement

Writing a personal statement is like applying for the job . You need to imagine what the job description might be for a medical student. You might expect them to be;

Interested in and have an understanding of medicine
Able to cope with the challenges that it will present.
Self-motivated and able to set and work to your own and other's deadlines.
Capable of working well in a team and on your own.
Have IT skills or be able to learn them.
Prepared to take all of the opportunities which higher education provides.
A great member of the university

Try to answer the following;

Why you have applied for medicine, what particularly interests you about it, any reading around the subject or relevant experience you have had, and any potential career plans.

Relevant school/college activities and awards or achievements and what you have gained from these.

Hobbies, work and interests .

Why you want to go to university/college

What you say is really up to you. But the difference between an ordinary and a special personal statement is planning. Sort out your thoughts, draft what you want to say, follow the advice below but take care to check spelling, grammar and punctuation.

The layout, content and style of your personal statement are your choice. Most people write in paragraphs but you can use sub-headings if you prefer. Do whatever you feel comfortable with but seek advice from school/college advisers, parents and friends before you commit yourself.

You may not feel that you have very much to say or that you have done anything of significance. Admissions tutors expect you to be able to reflect on what you have achieved and experienced. Parents may have a more positive view of what you have achieved so ask them.
Avoid making bland or incomplete statements, which just leave the reader with an unanswered question such as 'I enjoyed spending time at the radiology department' which begs the question 'why?'

So where do you start? Here are some thoughts;

What to do

Start early.
Be honest to yourself
Avoid redundancy when writing your statement
Be accurate about specifics, you will look foolish in the interview if you have exaggerated an achievement.
Make sure what you write is clear and grammatically correct
Remember each university will not know where else you have applied
Do it in a word processor.
Make sure it is not too long:
Cut and paste into the UCAS space to see if it fits
It is usually better to rewrite sentences rather than cut single words
Get lots of advice from the year above or friends, yours and your parents.

Try to attend open days particularly at schools you hope to be selected for. Try to speak to students, they are usually very approachable and friendly and give a useful insight into the pros and cons of the school. One family friend made a decision between two London schools on the basis of the 'feel' of the hospital bar!

Internet: but do not believe everything you read, students spending lots of time in fora may not be representative.

Some of the detail overlaps with the type of question you might expect in the interview. You may find ideal answers at the back of the book helpful when writing this section.

Areas you need to cover;

Why have you chosen to do medicine?

Make your reasons as specific as possible
Use anecdotes of what experiences made you decide
You can also acknowledge the 'down side' (hours, responsibilities…)
State what you have done to get better informed
For example you attended Medicourse and learned what?
Avoid clichés (helping people, making the world a better place)
It can be helpful to bring in science/art/humanities interface

What interests you about medicine?

Again, be specific and anecdotal
You can mention a specific patient or clinical situation
If you can, invoke an inspiring doctor you have known, as long as you can say why they was inspiring
You can mention medical articles you have read
It is good to mention challenges as well as positives
It is NOT good to mention salary!

Do you have any career intentions?

Your answer here must go beyond 'I am particularly interested in dermatology or psychiatry…' and say WHY
Invoke specific experiences within the speciality.
Don't be too rigid about choices – admit that you don't know enough yet to make an informed choice

Relevant work experience, placements and voluntary work

Don't restrict this to medical placements
Think about what might be relevant to medicine from experiences like,
Working in a shop
Helping out in a home for older people
Providing learning support in a primary school class
Be as specific as you can about medical placements you have done and what you have learned from them

Non accredited skills

Relevant items include
DoE awards, Young Enterprise, , Music
Emphasise what you have learned from the experience and why it is relevant to medicine

Social sports and leisure interests

Several medical schools pride themselves on exceptional sporting achievement and are on the look out for top sportsmen and women. You need to invoke, Achievement, Transferable skills, Ability to attain work/life balance
It is an opportunity to be genuinely self revealing.

Reasons for a GAP year

Good reasons include;

Becoming more mature and 'ready' for medicine
Doing something medically relevant
Learning new skills
Doing something useful
Less good reasons include;
A year of continuous partying or acquiring an Sexually Transmitted Disease….
Despite the reputation several schools actually encourage gap years that are well thought out.

Examples of personal statements

These are not designed to be copied but represent statements that have been well constructed and utilise the above advice. I have written in italics at certain points in the statements where a think a useful point is made. As you go through noting these points, think about them as you construct your statement.

Statement one

I have always wanted to be a doctor: all my experiences over the past three years have reinforced my strong belief that medicine is the career for me. I want to study medicine because I find the human body fascinating, I love biology and chemistry and I care passionately about people. I believe no other career brings these three aspects together more strongly, medicine is science with passion. (*reason for doing medicine, I like the last statement!*)

I am interested in Paediatrics: children often have a different perspective on life that I find stimulating. (*career intentions, supported with evidence*) During voluntary work at Kent and Canterbury Paediatric ward I formed a relationship with a 9 year old oncology patient, whose mother felt very comfortable leaving her daughter with me while taking a break from the hospital. We spent many hours playing games, having fun together.

To gain further insight into a medical career I organised various attachments. The first was to the Paediatric unit at William Harvey Hospital, Ashford, spending one week shadowing a Consultant and her team. I participated in ward rounds, outpatient clinics and admissions. I observed the importance of good teamwork and how doctors and nurses work together to benefit patients.(*using work experience to illustrate what she gained from the attachment*) I was surprised at the volume of paperwork involved (recognising the work implications). To provide experience beyond District General Hospital medicine I organised an attachment to a specialist hospital, Moorfield's. I was attached to Professor Bird where I observed in various eye clinics and attended early morning tutorials. Professor Bird is the most inspirational doctor I have ever met: I saw how having a strong leader directly benefits the entire team and the patients (*illustrating some of the values she thinks a good doctor might have*). In order to appreciate Primary care I have organised an attachment to a G.P. and will spend time with his Nurse Practitioner. I also subscribe to Student BMJ.

For the past six months I have visited Age Concern. With little entertainment available, I bought sets of dominoes and my arrival is eagerly awaited to play each week. I was delighted to be accepted onto the Millennium Volunteers Project, entailing 100 hours voluntary work at Kent and Canterbury Hospital which I will be commencing shortly (*not only work experience but evidence of considerable commitment*).

A defining moment for me was seeing children attempting to sharpen a tiny pencil, not much longer than one inch on the edge of what could barely be classed as a desk. I was on a trip to Kenya, which I personally funded and organised. (*interesting self organised and funded trip, evidence of what transferable skills were learned*) I travelled alone, stayed with a Kenyan family and taught English to a class of 79 Primary School children. I learned to think on my feet, to be resourceful and to quickly become independent in an alien environment – and I loved every minute of it! The Kenyan people made such an impact on me: I will never forget them. I learned that I can make a difference to other people's lives.

Having changed schools for the Sixth form, I felt it important to get involved in school life so I decided to take part in the annual school production which required teamwork, commitment and dedication (*again showing the skills learned rather than just what was undertaken*). I was proud to receive the Academic Effort Prize and to be invited to become a School Prefect with special responsibilities for integrating new pupils into the school (*nicely advertising leadership and academic skills in a non boastful manner*). I enjoy taking part in House sport matches within the school: although I am not a natural sportswoman I love the teamwork and friendly competitiveness involved. I have completed the Duke of Edinburgh Bronze Award, where leadership skills were highly important. I have taken part in several Maths Challenges, obtaining silver twice and a bronze recently.

I work in a pharmacy as a trained Medicines Counter Assistant. I am confident about asking people about their symptoms and recommending treatments (*more useful work experience with communication skills*). I find it very rewarding when patients return saying how they benefited from my advice.

In my free time I enjoy horse riding. I love the fresh air and having the freedom to switch off (*coping with stress*). I keep fit by regularly going to the gym.

My father has been the most influential person in my life. He has lived with MS for 17 years and has shown me how important it is to be determined, resilient and to not give up. I am hard working and I set myself high standards and always strive to achieve these. I have empathy with people and I have good communication skills. I am a team player, adaptable and versatile in all situations (*nice summary*).

Statement two
My interest in medicine has developed gradually over a period

of years; I had no eureka moment watching ER when I suddenly realised that I was going to be a doctor and that was final. Instead, my curiosity was initially sparked through conversation with my brother, who is now an F2. His obvious enthusiasm for his work was infectious (*evidence of an understanding of what it entails*). Though this greatly appealed to me, I knew I needed to ensure that I was well informed about the profession to see if it was right for me. At first, I attended work experience in a Minor Injuries Unit, shadowing a nurse practitioner. This was an intriguing, if hardly inspiring, first insight into medicine (*what not to write*!). I also attended a MediCourse, where I was given greater insight into the day to day life of a doctor and numerous specialities (*wise man, great course*!).

I have immensely enjoyed the opportunity to work with medical professionals and patients. As art therapist's aid on a stroke ward, I worked with recovering patients. Whilst I was aware that our contribution to their treatment was minor, I found it gratifying to see the small improvement that we could bring about in their dexterity, but most notably in their happiness (*interesting work experience giving an unusual insight*). I have also spent periods of time in an Endoscopy unit as a general busy body wiping down surfaces, making beds and brewing tea.

My most rewarding experiences have come working in an Alzheimer's care home and at a local hospice. The former, working as an RT's assistant, predominantly involved chatting with patients, walking them to the toilet and regularly being thrashed at dominoes; I also got involved in feeding and caring for the residents, generally trying to improve their quality of life (*nice work experience, not just following the professor on a ward round*). It was at the hospice that I really confirmed my interest in medicine. The insight into palliative care was eye opening, emphasising that medicine is about much more than curing patients; I left the hospice enthused by the genuine concern of the staff for their patients and their families (*again great experience and cannot be accused of not seeing the down sides to medicine*).

Despite the surroundings, their positivity shone through. It was a pleasure talking with these people and seeing them interact with their patients. I saw how worthwhile the role of the doctor can be, with the opportunity to make a genuine difference at all times, even in death. I know medicine is a challenging profession but I realised that it also offers a variety of experiences, consistently evolving, that will always provide new intrigue to me. Whilst it is based in science and this side is undeniably interesting, I believe that knowing the facts is barely a first step towards being a good doctor If that was it, the role would be little more than that of a technician. I believe that the profession requires so much more: most importantly, the ability to communicate and to empathise, both with patients and professionals from numerous specialities, whilst still providing the best treatment possible, whether this leads to a cure or not (*good reasons to be a doctor*).

I believe I am a confident, capable communicator, comfortable talking to large groups or in more intimate circumstances. Recently, I formed a company writing and performing murder mysteries for local fundraising events to rave reviews. This involves collaborating with fellow actors, keeping a large number of people in order whilst simultaneously creating an enthralling character. I always find drama a great escape with the opportunity to envelop yourself in a completely separate individual, and have performed in several local plays. I also make regular trips to the theatre, both at home and in London (*good evidence of team work and social skills*).

I'm currently a senior prefect, learning mentor and form guardian at my school (*leadership and organisational skills*). The grandiose titles aside, these are really organisational and disciplinary roles, where it's all important to earn the respect of younger students. There is a fair amount of responsibility attributed to these roles, and I work both with other pupils and teachers on a regular basis.

Whilst I am not the most talented sportsman, I am extremely keen to get involved where possible. (*If adequate space you might want to enlarge on how these activities contribute to your development as a person*) I regularly play tennis and table tennis to a fairly competitive level. I'm also a great film lover and go to the cinema whenever I find the time, devour books as often as I can get my hands on them and have recently taken up the theremin, despite being fairly tone deaf.

Statement three

I have become increasingly drawn to medicine by my curiosity about the human body and the scientific and technological aspects of medicine.
In the summer of 2004 I conducted a week's work experience at the John Radcliffe hospital. I spent much of my time in the wards, and really enjoyed talking to and helping the patients, as many of them appreciated having a friendly face (*good insight*). I was fascinated by the MRI scanner in the radiology department and the stunning images it generated.
In the surgery of a G.P., I saw the variety that exists within general practice and the close relationship between the G.P. and his patients. When shadowing a cardiologist at the Horton hospital in Banbury I was able to see the patients having tests that he recommended earlier (*might want to enlarge on this and say what it contributed to you*).
When I visited the clinical trials and services unit in Oxford, I found it exciting to be in a place where such influential discoveries had been made in the treatment of coronary heart disease and where Richard Doll's discoveries had taken place. The scale and precision of their investigations was amazing and I would like to participate in a research project at some point in the future.
At a Royal Society exhibition, I was intrigued by the possibility of a genetic test for coronary heart disease and the ethical and psychological implications of this. I am amazed at the way that the knowledge we now take for granted has developed, (*such as the process of vaccination*). I spent a week as a volunteer with Mencap, on a residential summer activity holiday for mentally handicapped adults, where I helped a lady with learning disabilities to participate

in both group and individual activities, as well as with personal care. Working with these adults made me realise how they can never become independent and made me think about the potential of gene therapy (*not bad*).

Over the last year I have achieved my 200 hour award as a Millennium Volunteer (*good stuff, real commitment*). I have taken out a 19 year old autistic girl, to help her have some fun and to spend time with someone her own age. It has been really rewarding getting to know and understand her, as I have learnt what to be aware of when being with her and how to recognise when she is happy (*that's the stuff*).

I love working with children and have been regularly baby-sitting and running activities at a children's holiday week in my village for a number of years. This year I have helped small groups of weaker swimmers during swimming lessons for the junior department of my school, and in running a French club for Year 8. This has allowed me to experience a certain degree of responsibility, and to share my enthusiasm for the subjects with others. I have also learnt how far a bit of encouragement goes, and how satisfying it is to see the students making progress and having fun (*now building up a picture of someone who has done a great deal of caring work with considerable responsibility*).

Spending a month in Bolivia with World Challenge was an amazing experience and I encountered many unfamiliar situations. At one point I found myself negotiating in Spanish with angry muleteers after a member of our team had collapsed. The trip proved to me the values of patience, tolerance and when leading the group, working efficiently as a team involves effective delegation and mutual trust.

When relaxing, I like to participate in a variety of sports and I love to read, both novels and books of general interest. I play tennis for both the school and my club, and hope to be a black belt in Tae Kwon Do in 6 months. I enjoy music and attend senior choir at school. I have almost completed my gold Duke of Edinburgh award (*what have these contributed?*).

From experiencing some of the huge variety that exists within medicine, I have become convinced that it is the area that I want to spend the rest of my life working in and feel that I could

Statement four

Throughout my life I have relished facing and overcoming challenges. I cope well with pressure, think on my feet, and work effectively both as part of a team and on my own. I am always dedicated to the task in hand, and believe that a career in medicine will allow me to excel and reach my full potential (*nice start, now prove it*).

Whilst spending time at each of Hinchingbrooke Hospital, in Trauma and Orthopaedics, and a local G.P.'s surgery, I observed the importance of 'bedside manner,' in addition to a doctor having the knowledge to diagnose a patient. They must have patience, and the ability to communicate effectively with a patient, to help them understand their condition and ensure they feel comfortable under their care (*good understanding of the role of the doctor*). I was commended for aiding younger pupils in mathematics at secondary school which required similar attributes, and hence I am confident I have the skills to make an excellent patient orientated doctor (*good*). During the coming year I will be working as a Ward Assistant at Addenbrookes hospital in Cambridge, and also intend to volunteer at a local residential nursing home.

Academically, Chemistry has given me a solid scientific knowledge, introducing many basic principles that I have found useful in other subject areas. I achieved the top mark for course work in my class demonstrating my ability in practical as well as written skills (*not sure I would put in too much about academic achievement unless it is extraordinary, they have details on your application form*). I have particularly enjoyed Human Biology, I am truly fascinated by the diagnosis of disease. For example, the use of monoclonal antibodies to test for glucose in urine as a preliminary test to identify whether a patient has diabetes or not. Advances such as these are making diagnosis rapid, accurate, and less invasive, hugely beneficial to the patient.

Maths has helped me with logical thinking and problem solving, whilst French has allowed me to explore a range of cultures from around the world, and has enabled me to read about a different approach to medicine, comparing it with our own (*yes, I like those explanations*). I also believe that it is essential to speak more than one language in today's world.

I am a keen sportsman reflected by the range of sports I enjoy. As well as playing hockey for Cambridgeshire Nomads on a regular basis, I am part of both the college tennis and hockey teams. I would hope to pursue these interests at university (*that might be helpful if they are looking for players*). I am excited by new challenges. Last year I obtained my PADI Open Water Diver, and I aim to become increasingly qualified in Scuba diving over the next few years. During the last year I have worked at 'Staples,' an office equipment retailer. I have very much enjoyed responding to customer's enquiries and solving their problems by finding a product to match their needs. The work has also included handling money and expensive items showing my trustworthiness (*fair enough but what about the communication skills needed to deal with difficult customers?*). I have also been involved in drama since my early teens which led me to perform at the Albery theatre in the West End, alongside Sean Bean, as 'Fleance' in 'Macbeth.' I have found my confidence has developed along with my communication and team playing skills. These are all transferable to the field of medicine (*great stuff*).

Throughout my AS year I have had to manage my time effectively, balancing study time, a job and my sport. This reassures me that I will be able to cope with not only the longs hours of medical school, but also the career ahead (*oh, yes, I like it*). I always take pleasure in hearing the developments in the medical profession, none more than a lecture by Doctor Michael Gaunt and his team at Addenbrookes hospital, on the use of ischemic preconditioning in dramatically reducing fatalities during the repairing of aneurysms. These events further enhance my desire to study and practice medicine, and I hope one day to make my own contributions to advancing patient care (*well OK, a bit specialised but at least he went*).

Statement five

My overwhelming ambition is to be a doctor I realise that it is a huge undertaking and is more a lifestyle than just a career but I believe that the reward will be a fulfilling and satisfying career. To be part of a team who have assessed and treated a critically ill patient I think must be a hugely rewarding experience (*nice introduction I think, its difficult not to be too gushing but it does give a lot of information in one paragraph*).
Equally, perhaps as a G.P. meeting young people and watching them develop and grow must be fulfilling and being able to contribute to their wellbeing must be a wonderful feeling. I also realise that there may be sad times as well as good times as I won't be able to help everyone but I believe that you can always help a little, even if it's just making their life more comfortable, holding their hand and listening to them (*good understanding of the down side of medicine and that palliative care can be as valuable as curative care*). I believe as a Doctor you have a great responsibility as people depend and trust you as a professional and I would be honoured to be given the opportunity for people to put their trust in me.
I attended an information day on osteopathy and physiotherapy. I have read various publications and have attended a Medicourse (*top effort, very shrewd*) where I was able to practice a number of clinical skills as well as gaining an insight into life as a student and as a qualified doctor and have decided this is the career for me.
I believe I have qualities which are essential for a career in medicine. I enjoy talking to all types of people and have been told that people find it easy to talk to me and that I am a good listener. People are happy to confide in me as they consider me trustworthy and discreet (*you might wish to illustrate this type of statement*).
To gain further insight into the world of medicine I work in an elderly people's care home where my duties include helping out at

meal times and also taking food to ill patients who cannot get out of bed (*good work experience, shows effort*). I also undertake cleaning duties. I enjoy chatting to the residents during my shifts and they seem to enjoy chatting to me.

I was lucky enough to be appointed as Head Boy of my House (*leadership*) during my time in Year 11. With this role I took part in public speaking at prize giving evening, and liaised between pupils and teachers on various aspects of school life. The role of Head Boy allowed me to develop my organisational skills and to further develop my negotiating skills (*great stuff*). I became a lot more confident both on a one to one basis and in a group, being able to make my point whilst also taking on board other peoples' views. My hobbies and interests include drawing, playing basketball for a national league team, swimming and reading, especially forensic science books.

I have gained many awards during my school life both academic and sporting. I have been privileged to receive an award each year at school prize giving and I have also received two trophies, one for commitment across the curriculum and one for service and sincerity (*bit nauseating but cannot fault the sentiment*). I found the awards motivating and encouraging. The service and sincerity trophy is awarded once a year to a pupil who has contributed to school, showing commitment and dedication during five years at secondary school. I was completely surprised to receive the service and sincerity trophy but felt very honoured (*modesty trophy a possibility too, but seriously, it is much better to come across as modest than arrogant*). When I was in primary school I swam in the Bazooka National Swimming Championships at Millfield School and my school came 6th overall. I have been swimming on a weekly basis since the age of four. My experience at the Championships made me proud of what commitment and dedication can achieve (*good*), I won all my races. As a further challenge I have enrolled on a National Pool Lifeguard Course later this year. This will enable me to combine swimming with learning life saving skills. I also enjoy rugby. I played for the Under 15's District Rugby Team. We competed in the District Championships and it gave me a true sense of being a team player (*that's the stuff*). We did very well and I made many new friends. It was a great opportunity to practice communication skills and to interact with people from all over the district. I hope you will consider me as a worthy applicant.

Statement 6

My first day as a Health Care Assistant, I remember walking in to the wards with a jumble of questions running through my mind simultaneously: Am I capable of caring for elderly? Will I enjoy it? (*interesting insight showing self awareness*) Within an hour these questions were given the answer I wanted as I busily cared for 25 patients at once. As I thought about how I had really enjoyed the whole experience of patient care and hospital work it gave me the knowledge that I am up for the challenge of a career in medicine. Along with the pleasure I take from building relationships with people, science has been a great fascination of mine. It is the endless possibilities that can result from the subject that makes it so appealing. This passion is what has primarily led me towards medicine. As I have grown and learnt I have been constantly astonished by the many diverse and complex systems of the human body.

Experience within the medical profession has affirmed my decision. When working in a home for people with dementia I learnt a great deal about the illness itself along with ways in which you can build relationships and communicate with the patients effectively despite their medical condition. I found this extremely rewarding, even when at times it could be challenging (*why was it challenging, what aspect*). With further research into Alzheimer's disease I found it to be a truly intriguing but yet devastating illness. In a two week period I spent shadowing a registrar A&E doctor in Southampton hospital I really got a feel for how both the hospital worked and the doctors within it. I not only realised the vast amount of knowledge and hard work that is required, but also the need for confidence in doctor's decisions and the patience that is constantly needed (*illustrating the qualities required*). It really allowed me to see all aspects of a doctor's career within the NHS, both good and bad. Such as the rewards of treating patients but the social sacrifices and paper work that will follow, or having the ability to help patients, but knowing that your help may not always be enough (*Good, shows an insight into the negative aspects of Medicine*). The opportunity provided me with a valuable perspective on hospital life and confirmed beyond any doubt that this is where my future lies.

This summer I have been employed as a health care assistant in Winchester hospital. I see this as the perfect way to prepare for a medical degree. It has shown the way in which hospitals are run from behind the scenes and has given me a great understanding about the NHS as an organisation. Caring and talking to many of the patients there has allowed me to build strong communication skills (*Good*). Even though it can be hard to provide palliative care for many patients, it has shown that I am more than able to deal with such difficult situations, which I know is such a necessity for a medicine degree and the career that follows.

As a keen traveller I have found myself back packing around Europe all summer, this experience has taught me much about establishing rapport with strangers in challenging situations. When exposed to many foreign cultures and languages I found a great desire to be able to communicate more effectively with many of the people. As a result I now find myself pursuiting to learn spanish in night classes. I plan to use much of the time I have this year by broadening my horizons in further travels. I believe will give an abundance of life experience and a more mature outlook on life as a medical student.

My dedication to sports has been life long with regular training sessions and matches for my local team in which I proudly own the captains band. This has led to me ensuring that all players including me, work as a team, which has vastly tested and progressed my leadership skills (*Team work and communication skills demonstrated*). The competitive side of me is brought out when playing past times such as golf and tennis in particular. I see sports as a way keeping both physically and mentally fit, and discovered it to be the perfect way to escape revision pressures during my A level period.

My dedication and perpetual desire towards the course has been illustrated through my second application, despite my disappointments from my unsuccessful application in 2006. With medicine I would relish the fact that I will never know it all, as there will always something new for me to discover. I hope to become a valuable member of a profession to which I truly aspire.

Statement 7

For me, a career in Medicine will allow me to explore my love of science, whilst constantly being faced with challenges and surprises. I have always been conscientious, so studying Medicine will give me the opportunity to combine this with my natural ability to empathise with others and my determination to directly help and succeed.

In December, I attended a 'PreMed' course which gave me an insight into the life of Medical students. It was particularly helpful to speak to doctors and I became aware of the benefits, but also the down side, to Medicine. I was eager to find out more so arranged work experience at a local Surgery where I was able to discuss issues with the doctors, talk to patients and carry out clerical work. This helped me to understand the workings of a General Practice and since then I have started reading the student BMJ, which had fuelled my ambition. To build up my skills, I attended a First Aid course and went on a residential 'Medicourse' during the summer. This was a particularly fulfilling and exciting experience and I had the chance to carry out an ECG and try suturing and taking blood, as well as going to lectures about various medical specialities. I became more aware of what a career in Medicine entails and feel that I have an acute understanding of what the years ahead of me will hold.

During Year 10, I worked in a nursery for two weeks, which made me far more confident and motivated me to take a more active role in my community, so I started to lead Sunday school for three and four year olds. I also helped with reading and science groups at a local primary school. I discovered that I enjoy being in a position of responsibility and that I work well with children.

Being a member of the 'Link Up' team, an organisation that works with children with disabilities, has taught me a lot about myself and although it has challenged me, (*good point scoring*) it has been thoroughly enjoyable. I now realise that these children value games and music as much as any other child. Their inability to communicate properly forced me to develop alternative ways of getting myself understood, enabling me to discover patience I never knew I had.

I currently volunteer weekly in a Residential Care Home, providing trolley service for the residents and spending time with them. I have gained a lot from doing this and despite being slightly apprehensive at first, I have realised just how friendly the older generation is.

In Year 11, I was History prefect and ran debate club for younger pupils. This challenged me, making me use my initiative and become more mature. I was part of the orchestra at secondary school and played on the netball team.

Besides my community and school work, reading and art are important to me, as is exercising. I frequently go to the gym and am quite involved in the Ruislip Rugby club community where I occasionally help in the kitchen. For me, my hobbies are just as important as the other things I do, as they give me time to reflect and unwind.

From the experience I already have, I believe that Medicine is a profession that will allow me to feel truly fulfilled and use all of my talents to their highest potential. Although Medicine is a demanding career, I know that it will be extremely rewarding to be making a meaningful contribution to society and so I look forward to the challenges I will face.

Statement 8

When I was 12 years old, I was admitted to hospital due to shortness of breath. This experience was very frightening and worrying to me and my parents. Nevertheless, I was astonished by the speed of my recovery and the normalisation of my breathing. This outcome made me immensely grateful to all doctors and nurses (*nice anecdote*). During this encounter and consequent follow-ups, I came to realise that a patient is not just a number, but a person whom everyone in the hospital handles with extreme care, devotion, sympathy, and respect. The way patients were systematically dealt with was very impressive. Doctors listened patiently and acted decisively on what they heard and observed. The care provided for by nursing staff was the most touching of all. During these visits, I became fascinated with medicine, the way diseases start and how they are treated and prevented.

During my work experience at Ninewells Hospital, Dundee I was able to shadow doctors on ward rounds and therefore got to see numerous patients suffering from various diseases, some of which were incurable. Furthermore, I had the opportunity to visit many departments including Paediatrics, Radiology, operating theatre and the Endoscopy Unit, which I found particularly interesting since it was an alternative to surgery and demonstrated a successful application of advanced medical technology. This unique experience gave me in sights into the enormous responsibility of the health services and stressed the necessity of the team work involved. I was particularly impressed by the work in the operating theatre as each one of the team, regardless of the tense atmosphere, found the time to teach junior surgeons. Observing the stream of practical knowledge flowing from senior to junior doctors was immensely encouraging. Living these moments of doctors in making, as they absorb live knowledge from seniors, had a profound impact on my career choice (*illustrates that he genuinely observed what was going on*). I came to realise that medicine is not only about making the correct diagnosis or providing the proper treatment, but also passing fundamental knowledge to future generations of young doctors. Living the spirit of hospital life at Ninewells hospital convinced me that medicine is the path I wish to follow for my career.

Taking part in extracurricular activities as much as possible is paramount in my college days. For example, I play football for the college team on a weekly basis. Playing football has taught me that team work is essential to win a game. Participating in sport is also stress reducing and helps me to cope with the immense amount of work involved in A levels. Living my early years between the Middle East and the United Kingdom gave me a unique opportunity to be exposed to different cultures. This was a learning experience as well as a chance to cross barriers and to encounter different cultures. The mixing of cultures in my early years not only promoted my confidence and sharpened my communication skills, but also made me appreciate how valuable it is to live in a multi cultural society like the UK.

Due to the large number of applicants, I was not fortunate to secure a place to study medicine. Consequently, I decided to have a gap year and reapply for medicine next year. During the gap year I will be part of a team (SENSE SCOTLAND) who work with children and adults across Scotland that need support because of deaf blindness or sensory impairment, physical, learning or communication difficulties. Other duties will involve assisting with bathing, dressing and personal hygiene. Working as part of a team will help create an ordinary living environment enabling people to use services to develop the skills they need to live an independent a life as possible. Focusing on communication I will encourage people to express their wishes and make informed choices about their lives with the dignity and respect enjoyed by other members in society. I understand that to succeed in these demanding, but rewarding roles, I will need to be flexible, responsive and able to deal with a changing environment.

Regardless of the fact that both my parents are doctors, I have tried to get the best idea of what it would like to be a doctor without being persuaded or influenced by their career choices. I came to realise that doctors must have the ability to act and react sensibly under pressure, as well as requiring experience, knowledge and skill in order to make the correct diagnoses and offer precise treatments.

I am a self motivated, determined individual and I look forward to the social and academic challenges of studying medicine. I am aware of the social sacrifices of a medical career and the continual academic commitment required, but my commitment and desire to become a doctor has only been strengthened through my work experience and academic aspects. By studying medicine I will not only help others, but pursue a career that I truly aspire. I believe that I would be able to meet the challenge and the stress of studying medicine and I sincerely hope that you will offer me the chance to prove myself. (*A nicely constructed statement making many of the points required*)

Statement 9

My passion for medicine stems from the research that I have carried out in exploring this exciting course and profession. I strongly feel an affinity towards medicine as it fulfils my desire to study the intricacies of the human body as well as allow me to help other people by using this knowledge.

I have been influenced by the medical field from a very young age as my uncle and aunty are both doctors. Talking to them about their work has increased my interest in the field and has led me to do further research and work experience in the local community and NHS (*you might wish to expand on why it increased your interest what do they do, what did they say?*).

My work placement at Newham Hospital proved extremely informative and enjoyable. I shadowed many doctors at different levels and also worked with the administration staff increasing my awareness of the NHS system and how it functions. In addition, I saw many endoscopies, observed doctors on ward rounds on a daily basis and talked to patients in order to gain an understanding of how they see the situation and how that differed from the doctor's viewpoint. This experience allowed me to gain a fuller understanding of the rigorous training and hard work that is required to be a doctor

In the microbiology department at King George Hospital I increased my awareness of the different diseases and the pathogens that cause them. I also gained the essential understanding of how the microbiology department is associated with the rest of the hospital. I used this opportunity to observe how the team works by spending time in all sections of the department from where the agar medium is made to where it is used to grow and observe the growth of different bacteria.

Every Wednesday afternoon in the past year, I have been in charge of organising and leading a sixth form team to help Year 5 students from local primary schools carry out various scientific experiments such as heart dissection and chemical tests. It allowed me to develop my ability to explain complicated scientific concepts logically and coherently to students of a younger age without using jargon. This experience also helped in developing my leadership skills.

Teaching a class of children at a local language centre allowed me to broaden my communication skills as I learnt to talk to a group as well as individuals. I attended staff meetings and talked to parents on their child's progress. This increased my confidence and prepared me for thinking on my feet, as I had to be ready to answer questions on a regular basis. I believe that my teaching experience will be very useful in delivering information to patients and relatives as well as other doctors.

A four day Medlink course at Nottingham University helped me to reinforce my decision to study medicine whilst increasing my knowledge in many of the different branches within medicine.

It also provided me with the exciting opportunity to watch a live operation by a video link where the patient's condition was explained beforehand. I also visited Medicourses recently and was able to practice a number of clinical skills including intubation, suturing, looking in eyes and ears and listening to abnormal heart and lungs sounds.

Regularly reading the New Scientist, Biological Sciences and Chemistry review magazines (and more recently the BMJ) has allowed me to maintain a growing interest in science..

Having joined the Duke of Edinburgh scheme, I have met new people and also enjoyed working as part of a team on the expedition part of the award. I have also learnt a great deal about team work from playing cricket in the Western Union Cricket League. It has taught me to think as a part of one team rather than an individual player.

I am certain that medicine is the only career for me as I strongly believe in hard work, determination and self improvement. I strongly desire to help others through my knowledge and learning. (*A good mix of work experience, reading and social and sporting activities*)

Statement 10

I first thought seriously about a career in medicine while working part time as a receptionist in a General Practitioners' surgery while studying for my A levels. I became interested in health care and was able to gain first hand experience of working in a medical environment. This led to me being able to sit in on some of the clinics and accompany the practice nurse on visits to local residential homes during the annual influenza immunisation programme. I also attended ante natal and children's clinics. As a receptionist I came into direct contact with patients and learnt to deal with their worries and concerns in a confidential and professional manner.

My father, a G.P., has been a consistent role model to me. He makes a positive impression on all who meet him, carrying out his role with compassion and expertise. His advice has been invaluable and his encouragement to take on work experience has been important for my own development. Through talking to him and other doctors at the surgery I realised how fulfilling a career in medicine could be, combining science, caring, working in a team and personal growth (*clearly has an idea of what she is undertaking*).

After my A levels I took a GAP year before university. During this time I spent two months working in India attached to a UK based charity, Health For All. I worked with a health team promoting a health and education programme in villages in Bihar, India's poorest state (*really interesting work and likely to be mentioned at interview, try to spot these 'stand-out' paragraphs and prepare to speak about them*). I experienced working with women's groups, addressing health issues such as contraception and the spread of disease and became familiar with common conditions such as malnutrition and malaria. I also spent time attending some of the village schools and helped teach English to the students. After my time in India I continued my travels for a further four months, having fun in Laos, Cambodia, Vietnam and Australia!

For the past two years I have been studying Psychology at the University of Sussex. I have enjoyed many aspects of the course and ended this year by attaining a high upper second class and believe I will ultimately achieve a first class honours degree. I would like to continue as a postgraduate and study medicine. I have particularly enjoyed the parts of the course related to human biology and medicine. As well as studying the biological bases of mental disorders and clinical and health psychology, my empirical project for my final year will involve researching post traumatic stress disorder after health events, particularly childbirth, cancer and cardiovascular disease.

While at university I have started working as a carer in the community for Caremark. I assist elderly patients in the community with domestic and personal care, enabling them to maintain their quality of life and have maximum independence in their own homes. My principal responsibilities include assistance with feeding, bathing and toileting and getting dressed (*good quality work experience*). I'm also involved in non physical care such as advice and encouragement and as a carer offer emotional and psychological support. I have worked independently in patients' homes, as well as communicating effectively with a team of other carers, to ensure high standards of professional care. I feel that I have gained first hand clinical experience and learned that teamwork, patience and empathy are vital when dealing with patients. My personal interests include travel, sailing and sport. At school I captained my school netball team and organised an out of school team in the Canterbury Women's League. I am a member of the university netball and ski clubs. I have recently started crewing on yachts and hope to be able to develop this activity. I am fully committed to a career in medicine. My experiences in caring, my enjoyment of the intellectual demands of my psychology degree and my ability to work as part of, and, when needed, lead a team, has convinced me I am ready to pursue the demanding path of a rewarding career in medicine.

A collection of personal statements is available, free, at http://thestudentroom.co..uk/wiki/Category:Medicine_Personal_Statements. This site also offers advice and some useful links to the various medical school listed in this book.

Chapter 2

Interview advice
Pre-Interview Preparation
General Advice
Body Language
Interview Structure
The Video
Ethical Scenarios
Inevitable questions

Interview advice

Different schools deal with the interview process in different ways, some have a panel of two, others much larger panels. Others include a student on the panel. For some you will complete a form prior to interview asking you some of the common questions such as 'why you want to be a doctor'. Others will provide an ethical scenario for you to read prior to being asked about it in the interview. Some like the Oxbridge colleges will ask academic questions almost to the exclusion of all others, most will want to know more about you as a person and what you will offer the School.

Pre-interview Preparation

Recommended books and journals
The Totally Brilliant.....well you have that one already
The Insiders Guide to Medical Schools BMJ Books
StudentBMJ online www.studentbmj.com
New Scientist
BMJ
Scientific American

medical news
see section later in the book.

medical blogs detailing the lives of medical students throughout the country

http://imamedicalstudentgetmeoutofhere.blogspot.com/
http://angrymedic.blogspot.com/
http://shortwhitecoats.blogspot.com/

Other excellent sites;
http://www.medschoolsonline.co.uk/index.php?pageid=85

www.thestudentroom.com
www.medicalschoolforum.com
www.admissionsforum.net

General advice

This is not the time to make a statement in life!
The interviewers have taken the time and trouble to dress smartly and prepare well for the interview. If you do not, then do not turn up at all.
Smell, don't! That is avoid strong scents (do wash though!)
Avoid excessive make up
Avoid jewellery if male, minimalist if female, tongue studs will not impress.
Look professional on entering the room
Don't sit until invited
Don't slouch
Don't cross arms
When introduced make eye contact and say hello
Make eye contact with the questioner but also the other team when speaking
Close the door after you on the way in and out.
Make small gestures with one hand to make a point, if making a series of points count them out on one hand.
Avoid grandiose gestures
'Would you like to ask any questions?' No is fine unless you have a cracker. Try 'no thank you, I was able to ask a number of questions when I visited the medical school'
Nod to the panel and say 'thank you'
Exit via the correct door, closing it!
Ensure you read newspapers in the months leading up to the interview and note down
Express ideas clearly and coherently with reasoned argument
Spontaneous, don't over coach

Assess what personal qualities good doctors require and ways in which you have acquired and can demonstrate some of them. If you aim to become a surgeon, in particular, prepare to give examples of manual dexterity and good hand-eye coordination. In all cases, how do you switch off and 'chill out'? All medical staff need to do this.

Reflect on what you have learnt about yourself and about the medical profession from your experience in any voluntary or social work or work shadowing you have done in a caring or medically related environment.

Show a keen interest in medical science that goes beyond the requirements of your school or college level studies. Focus on a small number of these topics and do some reading and research. The same applies to topical medical issues and concerns, ethical issues relating to health care, issues to relating to health administration and the medical dimension of modern lifestyles. Also go over any detailed projects touching on medical science which you have completed or are working on at school, etc.

Do your home work on the training offered by your target medical school and the career paths for doctors. Particularly the type of course, the environment, extra-curricular activities. (see choosing a medical school) Consider also the wider reasons why you are applying to that particular university. Prepare questions on matters of concern or interest that are not already answered in the medical school or university's literature.

Body language

Some schools actively mark body language
Don't; touch your face, play with your hair, speak with your arms crossed.
Do; make good eye contact, appear confident, sit forward, open. Take a folder in to hold

Interview structure

This varies between schools
Pre interview you may be given a questionnaire and or dilemma/case study to read or complete

The Video

Several schools use a video of a consultation on which you are expected to comment, more of this later.

The Article

Some schools such as St Andrews, give you a scientific article, perhaps from New Scientist for you to read and later comment upon.

The Ethical Scenario

Many schools now use an ethical scenario in the interview process, either as a scenario provided prior to you going into the interview room or during the interview itself

When answering this question try to use the following structure and 'buzz' words.

Autonomy, the right of a patient to be involved in decision making which affects him or her

Beneficence, the importance of doing good

Non-malificence, the importance of doing no harm

Justice, in this context this relates to managing available resources for the maximum benefit of the population

I will deal with ethical scenarios later in the book but here is an example of how you might use these terms;

Question; Is it fair to offer an alcoholic a liver transplant?

We have guidance from the GMC that indicates that we should not deny medical care to people on the basis that their disease is selfinflicted. The patients autonomy needs to be respected, they should be involved in decision making with regard to their health and we should be non judgemental. We should not offer treatment likely to do harm but have to balance risk with benefit. A liver transplant is a major procedure carrying a significant mortality and so we have to balance this risk with the probability of improving quality of life and longevity. If the patient is still drinking this will increase health risks and diminish the likelihood of benefit. With regard to justice, we have to make decisions, guided by NICE and by Primary Care Trusts as to how the available budget should be used for the maximum benefit of the population served. It might be considered that on this basis the benefit of a liver transplant in an alcoholic might not warrant denial of an alternative treatment of a cancer sufferer

Inevitable questions

Why choose medicine?

The most rehearsed and predictable question
Not 'because I want to help people'
Why DO you want to be a doctor, does one speciality fascinate you.
Why not a nurse, vicar, policeman?
What are the negative aspects?

Why at this school?

Have a good understanding of the course

Problem based learning, what are the pros and cons
Why this school, what are its pros and cons. Why a new school?
What in the prospectus appealed to you?
Try, I found the training program well constructed in comparison with others I had looked at and it offers an early opportunity to begin clinical training
I find that PBL suits my style of learning
For larger teaching hospitals you might mention that because it comprises several hospitals it provides opportunities to experience teaching at several units

How do you cope with stress?

How do you cope with stress
How do you cope with situations where there is not enough time to finish a task?
How did you cope with the stress of the GCSEs
What do you do when you have 3 or 4 urgent tasks to perform?
Are you a leader or a team player? What are the duties of a leader

Previous work or caring experience

Facts and details
Emotional response
What it taught you
What you gained
What aspect of your work experience did you find most and least interesting and why
What aspect of your work experience would you recommend to a friend thinking about medicine and why?
What would you do differently at the hospital/practice you attended
What skills did you learn that you can apply to medicine

Depth and breadth of interest

You are expected to have an intelligent lay view of medical matters,

particularly those of current media interest.
What medical stories are significant in the media at the moment?
Tell me about a book or film that has influenced you and why

Contribution to Medical school

What would you like to be remembered for from your medical school life?
Which activities do you think you would like to do?
Would you like to continue your pole dancing or would you do something new?

Topical subjects likely to come up in the interview

Human cloning, tell me what the advantages and disadvantages of human cloning might be? (256)
Tell me about the problems related to obesity and how we might tackle obesity nationally (190, 208, 227)
Tell me about antibiotic resistance and its causes
What does NICE do? (204)
What do you know of stem cell research? (190)
What are the political parties doing to improve patient choice in the NHS (190, 208, 224)
EWTD (see page 238)
'Payment by results', Practice Based Commissioning and 'choose and book' (see 190)
The Foundation programme and run through training (191, 203, 230)
Herceptin in breast cancer (190)
Cervical cancer vaccine 226, 231)
G.P. pay rises and out of hours.
Global warming see below

Recent Journal or newspaper items

The student BMJ and National electronic library for medicines (http://www.nelm.nhs.uk) are very useful sources of recent medical information.

Global warming and health (Telegraph online)

Flooding and drought with bring attendant health problems, "There are health effects secondary to flooding, such as contaminated water supplies, that could result in the spread of infectious diseases," he said.
Droughts, which are becoming more common and longer lasting, can lead to starvation and the destruction of entire ways of life, particularly in regions such as subSaharan Africa that are least equipped to deal with such catastrophes.
McGeehin also foresees the possible spread of mosquito borne illnesses such as malaria, dengue fever, yellow fever and encephalitis. "As the climate warms, we may see a change in the range of vector borne diseases," he said.

"In the very places where glaciers are retreating, we are also seeing a lengthening of the season of transmission of the disease in parts of Africa," Epstein added. In Africa, there has been an increase in Rift Valley Fever, which affects animals and people, as well as cholera, he said.
Epstein noted that even in the United States, ticks, mosquitoes and other insects that carry disease such as West Nile Virus, Rocky Mountain Spotted Fever, Eastern Equine Encephalitis and Lyme disease are already spreading to areas once considered too cold for them to survive.
In addition, increasing air pollution from the continued burning of fossil fuels will cause higher rates of respiratory and cardiovascular disease, McGeehin said.
"With warming, there are also increases in pollen and mould spores," Epstein added.

Hay fever vaccine in a pill http://www.nelm.nhs.uk

The first vaccine pill for hay fever sufferers will be launched in January 2007 reported seven newspapers (12 December 2006).
The reports appear to be based in part on a news item on the MRC website. It is not possible to comment on the reported trial results as we have been unable to identify the source of the information.
Seven newspapers reported on a new hay fever treatment, Grazax, the first treatment targeting pollen allergies to be available as a pill. It contains Timothy grass pollen extract that causes a protective immune system response. The pills dissolve under the tongue and need to be started two months before the beginning of the hay fever season.
Most papers reported that in trials, patients receiving the pill reported a 30% reduction in symptoms such as itchy eyes and sneezing; a 40% reduction in the need for other medications; and 80% of patients felt better after taking the tablets. Some of the reports pointed out that the pills will only be prescribed to patients for whom existing treatments are ineffective.
The newspaper articles appear to be based in part on a news item on the MRC website . Despite extensive searching it has not been possible to identify the source of the trial results reported. A five year trial assessing the long-term effects of the treatment is currently ongoing.

"Blood test that predicts strokes or heart attacks" http://www.nelm.nhs.uk

A simple blood test can predict a heart patient's risk of serious illness or death reported four newspapers (10 January 2006). In general, the reports accurately summarised the results of a well conducted study that found that blood concentrations of a protein called NTproBNP were related to cardiovascular risk in a large group of heart disease patients.
The reports are based on the results of a well conducted study of 987 people with stable coronary heart disease who were followed

up for an average of 3.7 years. This looked at the association between a range of factors measured at the time of study entry and the subsequent rate of cardiovascular events and deaths. The results suggested that participants with the highest blood concentrations of a particular protein called NTproBNP were over 3 times more likely to have a cardiovascular event that those with the lowest concentrations.

The main factors of interest were those that might predict death or cardiovascular events, with a particular focus on NTproBNP. The range of baseline NTproBNP concentrations was divided into quartiles to allow comparisons between groups of patients.

What were the findings?

Individuals with NTproBNP concentrations in the highest quartile had an almost 8-fold increased rate of cardiovascular events or death than those in the lowest quartile. After adjusting for other factors, a 3.4-fold increased rate of cardiovascular events or death remained in the highest quartile compared to the lowest quartile.

The addition of NTproBNP level to standard clinical assessment and findings from echocardiography resulted in a statistically significant increase in the ability to predict adverse cardiovascular outcomes.

What were the authors' conclusions?

The authors concluded that NTproBNP level is a predictor of adverse cardiovascular events among ambulatory individuals with stable CHD, independent of other prognostic markers. They suggest that level of NTproBNP may help guide risk stratification of high risk individuals, such as those with CHD.

Cost effectiveness of statins for vascular disease http://www.nelm.nhs.uk

Widening the use of statins, beyond current guidelines to people at low risk of heart attack or stroke, could be beneficial reported three newspapers (10 November 2006). The papers gave an accurate summary of a cost effectiveness study, though the model had limitations that should be considered when interpreting the findings.

Three newspapers reported that individuals with a 1% risk of heart attack or stroke, who are as young as 35, could benefit from taking statins to lower cholesterol. Two reported that the cost of prescribing statins for people at lower risk than currently receive this medication was less than the cost of caring for patients who have a heart attack or stroke.

The newspaper articles are based on a cost effectiveness model The researchers extrapolated data from a randomised controlled trial of patients with heart disease or diabetes comparing the drug simvastatin to placebo for an average of five years. They used the data to develop a model assessing the lifetime cost effectiveness of taking statins and the cost effectiveness of using the drug with older and younger age groups and people at lower risk of disease than those included in the RCT. The authors concluded that treatment with statins is cost effective in a wider population than is currently routinely treated based on current UK guidelines.

HIV testing (Student BMJ)

The UK government has made it a policy priority to increase uptake of HIV testing and is funding prevention programmes in England for the population groups most at risk. Services throughout the country offer voluntary testing, confidential partner notification, and education and support for affected people and their partners. These measures rely on a crucial relationship of trust and confidence between patients and health care professionals.

The sustainability and success of this approach are threatened by the policy of criminal prosecution. Although people with HIV or at risk of infection have had many reasons to be fearful about the impact of HIV, the possibility of appearing in a court of law followed by imprisonment had not until recently been one of them. But 2001 saw the first successful prosecution in Scotland for "reckless injury," followed by some in England and Wales for "reckless transmission" of HIV, under the Offences Against the Person Act 1861. The Terrence

Higgins Trust, a UK HIV charity, says more cases are in the pipeline.

Already this use of the criminal law is having unintended negative consequences. Awareness is spreading in people with HIV that they face the threat of criminal prosecution. Media coverage has vilified convicted people as "AIDS assassins," exacerbating the stigma already associated with infection. No wonder people unlucky enough to become infected often choose to keep their status a secret.

People in this situation need help and support to plan how and to whom they will disclose their status, and to find strategies for protecting other people from infection. With a spouse or long term partner, suddenly refusing to have sex or requiring the use of condoms without explanation is unlikely to be effective. But disclosure of HIV status may lead to rejection, physical violence, and financial destitution.

If word gets out into the community, perhaps through a sexual partner, people with HIV risk being ostracised, with their families taunted and their employment and entire existence under threat. Health professionals can advise and help, but their patients, if fearful of prosecution, may be unwilling even to tell them if they are having difficulties avoiding unprotected sex.

Who infected whom?
An estimated 200000 people in the United Kingdom have HIV infection that is still undiagnosed. There is a clear disincentive to testing when prosecution relies on defendants knowing they are infected. Meanwhile, people who take the test may not agree to their partners being notified for fear of legal repercussions, thereby jeopardising essential efforts to control public health. In addition, the threat to the confidentiality of data posed by criminal investigations may deter participation (or honesty) in the sexual behaviour research that provides an essential evidence base for HIV prevention. Doctors need guidance on whether the potential for criminal prosecutions changes their legal and ethical duty of confidentiality

and how to advise their HIV positive patients, who may become "victims" or "defendants" if a prosecution occurs. A draft briefing paper can be obtained from the British HIV Association.

Evidence on the impact to public health of criminal prosecutions for reckless transmission of HIV is limited, and further research is urgently needed. Uptake of HIV testing in groups at highest risk should be monitored to see whether criminalisation may be leading to reductions.

In England and Wales, the draft policy on criminal prosecution for the "sexual transmission of infections that cause grievous bodily harm," states that a prosecution will usually take place "unless there are public interest factors tending against prosecution which clearly outweigh those tending in favour." Putting aside the difficulties in attributing who infected whom, we would argue that, in the case of criminal prosecution for reckless transmission of HIV, the public interest is not best served by pursuing justice against the few at the expense of the health of the man

Remind yourself why you want to become a doctor

Before your interview, scrutinise your UCAS form and be expected to be asked questions on anything you have put down if you lie on it then you've got a good chance of being found out . Talk about what you had gained from your experiences mentioned on your UCAS form rather than just reeling a list off of what surgical procedures you have seen. You could also try to link your experiences to something you have read about in journals/newspapers recently if you're feeling really clever.

Practising

Practice with anyone: parents, teachers, siblings, friends, They are invaluable in informing you about your body language and eye contact, You can check you progress and watch whether you come across well to the interview panel.

The interviewers will always find new questions so be prepared for anything and think broadly. Do not sound as though you're reading from a script or over rehearsed.

The difficult question

If you get a question which defeats you. It is probably designed to do so. They are looking for people who think 'outside the box' and have an interesting take on a question such as 'how would you spend the NHS budget?' If you really have no idea 'name five types of arthritis associated with psoriasis', admit defeat gracefully and move on. If you manage to get some brownie points later in the interview then the assessors will probably forget about the first incident.

The pre-interview video

Several medical schools now show a video of a consultation and ask you to comment upon it.

There are many books on the consultation and many consultation models of varying complexity. They tend though to follow either the medical model whereby the doctor asks closed questions such as 'have you passed any blood in your urine' aiming specifically to confirm or exclude a diagnosis or the patient centred model as outlined below. The important features of the patient consultation as outlined by the Royal College of General Practitioners include;

Does the doctor allow the patient to contribute?

Does he pick up on cues, that is body language or words that suggest an underlying concern. Such as 'I have had a headache for four weeks. I thought I had better see you as my granny had a brain tumour'

What are the social or psychosocial factors, that is, what factors at home or at work might be influencing their illness. An example would be the lady that comes depression and reveals that her husband is abusing her.

Explores the patients health understanding, that is, asks the patent what they think is wrong. This might seem odd to the layman but it can reveal an underlying anxiety that one would never have thought of otherwise. A man cam to see me with several swellings under his skin, lipomas, benign fatty lumps. I explained what they were and he was hugely relieved and revealed that he was convinced they were cancer and he had been putting off coming for weeks because he was convinced I would confirm his imminent demise.

Excludes or confirms significant disease, you would not be expected to comment on a diagnosis without training.

Explains the diagnosis in terms that are understood by the patient and confirms that the patient understands the explanation.
Involves the patient in management decisions.
Prescribes appropriately
Encourages compliance , that is provides information and reassurance about the treatment offered in an attempt to ensure the treatment is taken.
Arranges follow up.

You are likely to wish to comment upon the body language displayed, the involvement of the patient and whether you think their concerns have been addressed or explored

Chapter 3

Sample medical school interviews and information
A collection of questions previously used in interviews
General Tips on the Interview

Sample medical school interviews and information

I have collated over 100 medical school interviews largely from Medicourse attendees, some of which have also been posted on web sites, I thank everyone who has contributed. Most medical schools provide some general information on their websites for prospective candidates, some like HYMS publish previous questions on their site. I have included some of the more typical information along with reported interviews.

St Andrews, The University of, Faculty of Medical Sciences

St Andrews give you an article to read and summarise the main points.

Interview 1
Why medicine?
Why St Andrews and Manchester?
What did you learn from your work experience?
What are some of the difficulties with being a doctor
They really focus on your personal statement,

Interview 2

Why St Andrews,
Why medicine,
Questions on the personal statement
Then they move on to asking me about the article. Mine was on methods of cheating in sports but you don't need to have any previous knowledge of the topic at all! It was from New Scientist and was simple to understand, you really just need to be able to remember and summarise the main points, you are given plenty time to read it

Barts and the London School of Medicine and Dentistry

Interview 1
I see you live near Barts, I bet you're annoyed we called you to interview at The London.
Video related questions What in your opinion makes for a good doctor
What effect can poor communication have on professional relationships. Do you think such issues impact on patient care?
As a doctor you will have to explain complex procedures to lay people. Imagine I am that lay person and tell me about your doctoral research.
What are you currently reading?
What appeals to you about BL?
What do you do to relax? Why do you think we asked you that?
What student activities do you think you would like to get involved with if we made you an offer?
I see from your university history, you are an impressive candidate. What happened at A-Level?
Followed by 'Oh! Um! You don't need to tell us about this if it makes you feel uncomfortable'!
Then a little bit of random chit chat about life at that time...

Interview 2
Mature student interview
Why Barts?
Why now in a nutshell?
When was I in Africa?
Why did it take me so long to act on my decision?
Asked about my kids
Are any of them thinking of doing medicine?
What did I do in my voluntary work? Working with younger students
Duration of course + training G.P.
What company I worked for What I was doing on Project (health, safety, environmental)

Gave an example of hydrogen sulphide toxicity and sulphur dioxide respiratory, ambient air quality, modelling detechnalised
What I thought of A levels in the 70s Vs now?
How did I find them?
Low morale and doctors
Why 5 year and not 4 year course (no pure science degree or bio science background)
What would I do hockey, most probably mixed and refereeing
Asked medical student what she did discussion on fencing
What did you do on your work experience at hospital?
Who organises patient treatment at a hospital? What did you learn?
What did you learn at G.P.'s?
What differences are there between a G.P.'s and consultants role?
Which position involves more teamwork?
How is teamwork important in a G.P.'s/ in a hospital?

Interview 3
How did your work experience help you make the decision?
What part of a doctor's life made you decide that medicine was for you?
In a team who is the leader?
You are very actively involved in your present university's extracurricular activities, what will you bring to Barts?
Tell us about your final year project?
What implications does this have for medical students and what are the strategies coming from the results?

Interview 4
 What did I think of consultation
 What qualities are needed in a doctor
What qualities do I have that will make me a good doctor
What I "took away" from my work experience
What scares me most about being a medical student
What story in the news is of interest to me…
What I thought of video
What I can contribute

My work experience
Problems of being a doctor
Why I wanted to be a doctor
Mine was very quick 10 min. but some people were there for 20?

Interview 5
How was your journey.
What did you think about the video? What good and bad things did he do? What would you do differently if you were in that position?
Tell me about Russell Silver Syndrome. Did this inspire you to do sign language?
Talk about your work experience. What were the demographic differences in the G.P.'s surgery and at the urologist.
If I gave you £10000 to spend on a gap year, what would you do? Why?
What proportion of your time should you spend relaxing compared to working? How do you relax?
Talk about an article you read recently.
Why Barts?
When did I first become interested in medicine?
What qualities does a doctor need?
Advantages and disadvantages of being a doctor
How would I cope with disadvantages?
Why Barts?
What did I witness on my work experience?

Interview 6
If I had to write a person specification from a patients point of view what qualities would I like a doctor to have? What about trust?
If I was to try and put someone off a career in medicine what would I say?
If an ambulance brought a friend into hospital and I was a fourth year student attending on placement what would I do? What about if I was a G.P and they came in and collapsed in my practice?
Why Barts? Why is there a wealth of clinical experience in this area?
What did I do and learn during my work experience?

What have I been doing since I left school two years ago?
What is it about being a doctor that attracts you?
How was your journey?
You saw the video; do you have anything to say about it?
Anything you thought the doctor did wrong / right
What do you think the patient may be worried about?

Interview 7
Why Barts?
Any good points about medicine?
Any bad points about medicine?
How do you cope with stress?
Apart from art and literature, what other hobbies do you have?
Any sports?
What would you take part in here at Barts?
When did you first hear about this university?
Why are computers so great?
 Did you come down today or travel last night? How was your journey?
 You saw the video, what was your overall impression of the consultation?
 Have you been around the campus etc? What do you think of here?
Tell us what you know about pbl...
 If you wanted to put someone off studying medicine, what would you say?
Can you tell us a little about what you do in your voluntary work in A&E?
What is it you have learnt from all your work experience?

Interview 8
I presume you took the train down, how was your journey?
Questions about the video what did the doctor do wrong or right
What are the downsides of medicine?
Reading anything at the moment? Literature?
What do you do to de-stress?
Is there anywhere you can play the violin without annoying anyone

else?
Why Barts
Read about any recent ethical medical issues?
What exactly happened
DO you think the medical staff could have handled it any better?

Interview 9
What did I think of the video?
What are the negative aspects of becoming a doctor
What do I read?
Talked about History A-Level and then asked me how American Foreign Policy has changed over the years.
What were the main reasons in Nazi rise to power?
Why Barts?
What do I do to relax?
What was the most influential lesson I learnt from my work experience?
If I was given £20,000 what would I do with it.

Interview 10
How was your journey?
How would I build rapport with patient
What qualities am I looking for on my G.P.
How can the G.P. achieve trust
Asked about history of Barts, more specific on William Harvey
Why Medicine
About hobbies
Why I have the hobbies that I have
Disadvantages of being a medical student and later a doctor
What made me decide to change profession

Interview 11
How was your journey?
What did you think of the consultation (video)? What do you think you would have done?
What did you learn from your work experience? What did you learn

there which made you want to be a doctor What negative aspects did you see?
What can you offer Bart's?
Why Bart's?
If you were to discourage someone from being a doctor, what would you say?
"Today I had a patient who was due for a kidney dialysis but was being totally despondent, not talking and that... she was meant to have it a month back but refused and now her health has really deteriorated. All her family want it done. Would you go ahead and give her the treatment?"

Interview 12
On the video.. If you were the G.P. in the video would you do anything different? If so what? And Why?
Questions on Autism... (I did some volunteering at an autistic school and put this on my personal statement that's why they asked about it!)
Why a doctor and not something like a physiotherapist?
Why should we pick you?
Have you looked at the prospectus and what do you think of the course structure?
What clubs/societies would you like to join at this university?
What are the difficulties of being a doctor
How do you relax?

Interview 13
We had to watch a 5 min. tape about a G.P. patient consultation, and were asked questions about it in the interview.
What did you think of the G.P. behaviour in the consultation?
How could he improve it? What would you require of a doctor
What clubs/societies would you join?
What is the problem around this area?
What are the benefits of studying medicine in such an area?
Explain the structure of studying medicine here?
What are the benefits of PBL?

Why Queen Mary's?

Interview 14
Questions about the video.
What are the bad points of becoming a doctor
What are the implications of those points you mentioned?
What are differences between the skills of a G.P. and a hospital doctor
Why did you put Barts down on your ucas form?
Why did you choose to study religious studies?
What are the ethical issues that arise from stem cell research and cloning?
What kind of illnesses are more common in the east London area?
What can you bring to this medical school?
You've done a lot of things in your spare time, how did you manage to fit it all in?
Do you have any questions?

Interview 15
Why us?
Why do you think PBL prepares you for professional life?
What are your hobbies outside of school?
What did you think of the video?
What skills/qualities do you have that make you think you would be a good doctor
Have you had any work experience where you saw something which made you think about your future as a doctor For example, something you would like in the future?

Interview 16
What did you think of the video?
Was the lady happy?
What qualities should a doctor have?
Do You have these qualities?
What do you know about the course at Barts?
Tell us about the work experience at the hospital

Tell us about the Fordway Centre
What do you like about Barts?
What would happen if you didn't communicate well with a patient?

Interview 17

Questions concerning the video
Asked to compare diseases in the third world and the first world were very keen on cardiovascular problems
Wanted to know what risk factors were involved in obtaining TB in the east end and a general discussion of diseases in the third world and that of the East end?
Asked if I was put off by medicine by any of the doctors I undertook my work experience with.
What qualities are needed in a doctor
Finally, what can I contribute to the medical school
Duration was approx. 15 mins

Interview 18
Have you heard on the human genome project?
What ethical issues have you seen or heard about recently?
The interviewer put forward an argument for Euthanasia and asked me to briefly argue against it.
What do you think will be at the cutting edge of medicine in 20 years time?
If you could wave a magic wand and cure one illness or disease in the world what would it be?
You have worked with the elderly. What do you think it is like to be old?
What problems do the elderly encounter?
What do you think you could contribute to this medical school?
So, have you heard from anywhere else?
How are you going to choose between 3, or maybe now 4 medical schools?
What are the good qualities of a doctor
Medicine is a life long career, how do you think or which part of our

course structure will prepare you towards it?
Describe me your work experience
Tell me more about the problems faced in the NHS or give example of situations or problems in NHS you saw whilst you were doing the work experience
Do you read any medical journals or scientific journals such as The BMJ or The New scientist? If so, tell me more about an article you read recently
Did you come for the Open Day?
If so, you probably know more about the clubs and societies that we have, which ones would you join?

Interview 19

What qualities are looked for in a doctor and how do you have them? / If you were a patient what qualities would you expect your Doctor to have?
I see you've done a lot of work experience what have learnt from all this?
Have you ever been in conflict with someone? How did you deal with this?
What would you do/say if someone disagreed with what you do regarding ethics.
I you were in A&E and a traumatic injury came in that a friend was involved with, how would you react/deal with this?
What do you know about the course at Barts (read the prospectus cover to cover, luckily I did that this morning)
I see you live in the east end, what problems are associated with the area?
We like well rounded individuals at Barts, how will you contribute to the school?
What have you done to find out about a medical career?
Describe an ethical issue in the news lately and your view on it
What diseases do rich people have?
Which ones do poor people have?
Why is Tower Hamlets a deprived area?

Tell me about your Young Enterprise Co.?
Would you not rather be a high flying business person?

Interview 20

What happened last year (I'm retaking)?
What are the qualities of a good doctor What do you think of your doctor do you visit regularly?
What is the most unpleasant thing about being a doctor
What will worry you most as a junior doctor
What are the advantages of being a G.P. over a surgeon. Have you though about general practise?
What are the health problems associated with the East End?
How do you think the language barriers here make it difficult for doctors?
What stood out to you on your work experience?
What negative publicity has the NHS had recently?
What hobbies will you bring to Barts? Will you try anything new?
What do you think of problem based learning. What are the pros and cons?

Interview 21

What do you see as possible problems in your future career.
What recent things in medicine have caught your eye.
What qualities are important for a doctor
Knowledge of teamwork aspects.
What you can bring to the college not only academically but socially
Why did you choose Queen Mary's?
Why do you want to study medicine?
What do you think are the qualities of a good doctor
What qualities do you have that would make you an ideal doctor
What are the main health problems in the East End?
Why do you think there are so many problems in the East End area?
Which aspects of the course at Queen Mary's particularly interest you?

What is problem based learning? What are the advantages of it?
What was the last article you read in New Scientist? (I got that
questions because I'd written in my UCAS form that I regularly read
New Scientist)
If you were a G.P., how would you monitor your patients' health?
Did you read the prospectus? What interests you about the area?
Are you planning on doing any more hospital based work
experience? If so, where?

Interview 22

What have you done to find out about medicine (as a career)?
What did I see while working with the surgical team? (during work
experience)
How did I find working with elderly people?
What problems would elderly people have with going into hospital
instead of to a day care centre?
What recent articles have interested you in biological science? (I said
about HIV and AIDS)
How will making people aware of HIV and AIDS make a difference
to the number of people affected??
Which medical scandals have interested me?
Discussion of what I did in my voluntary work on Renal unit/
medical ward and what I'd learned from it.

As a student who's that "little" bit older, what do you think you
could bring to the medical school and some of the younger students?
(Again in the context of being a mature student) Have you given any
thought as to what you might like to do? (Led to a discussion about
inner city health care problems/ epidemiology)
If people in the inner cities have more health problems and greater
health care needs, they should get the best care. Do you think this is
the case? (I said no)
Why not? (talked about financial causes, the private sector and also
awareness/ education about what options are available)
How do you think your previous (Arts) degree will help you in the

medical course?
Interview 23

Why I still wanted to do medicine after all this time
Disadvantages of a career in medicine
Work experience (only listed what I'd done, nothing deep)
Question's about my degree
Given my age, what did I have to contribute to the life of the medical school (clubs, societies etc)
How I'd fit in with mainly younger people
What graduates can bring to the course
Did I realise how much work / study it would entail
How was I finding A level chemistry
Financing myself
Was I taking the tour

Interview 24

Why QMW?
Why medicine?
Have your Doctor parents tried to discourage you?
Have they not suggested alternate careers for you?
Tell me about your work at ….
Tell me about your work on an Orthopaedic ward
What part of science do you like the most?
If you were given a ward with people with infection, how would you go out treating them?
What do you think about antibacterial wipes?
Tell me a bit about your travelling
What clubs/societies would like to join in the University?
Any questions?

University of Birmingham, School of Medicine

Similar format to HYMS, Birmingham had a larger panel, HYMS two. Interviewed in November, Offer in December

Extracurricular activities
What will you contribute to university life?
CV related questions largely

Brighton and Sussex Medical School

Why do you want to be a doctor
What do you know about the NHS?
About 10 years ago there was a great shortage of Bristish doctor's so many doctors were brought over from India to practice in the UK. What do you think about this?
Tell me about a medical breakthrough in twentieth century.
Why did you do a Psychology degree? Why didn't you apply to medicine instead?
What difficult situation have you experienced and how did you manage with it?
If you had a coat of arms what slogan would you put on it?
If you don't get into medicine this year what will you do next year?
Do you think it is important that the leader of a team is liked?
Tell me about an infectious illness you have heard about recently in the news.
After a long day at University do you find yourself wasting time in the evening?
What's your favourite film?
What skills have you learnt from your degree that will contribute to medicine?

Bristol, University of, Faculty of Medicine

Interview 1
Should have been 10-15 min. but I think it was longer. With a male G.P. and female university person. Interview in morning, tour in afternoon.

Where is Bicester (home)?

How long does it take you to get to school and how do you get there?
Why medicine?
Any particular area you think that you would like to go into?
Tell me about your work experience in the research place, describe what they were doing.
What are the worst things about being a doctor
How do you cope with pressure?
What are the challenges of working with people?
Can you give me an example of a time when you have been in a similar situation?
Tell me about something that you have read in the newspaper.
Do you know how vaccines work?
Ethical questions about cervical cancer vaccine, what age do you think it should be given and who should decide?
Any questions?

Interview 2

In my Bristol interview, they focused on the ethical and social sides of
medicine as a degree course as opposed to the science. They started with the
classic: why do you want to study medicine and why at Bristol? They asked me about the course structure and how clinical placement are arranged. We talked about what happens when you graduate (FY1,FY2, etc). They asked me about ethics and seemed impressed when I mentioned the four principles of ethics (autonomy, etc). I had done the DoE awards, so they asked me what I gained from them. They did not give the impression that they were trying to catch me out with tricky questions. The most unusual question was probably: could you sum up the DoE award in three words!
Two doctors and a medical student interviewed me. They really were very friendly, they did their best to put me at ease and did not seem at all threatening. They basically just wanted to chat to me to work out what I was like as a person.

Interview 3
Why do you think Bristol (as a city) would be a good place to study?
What problems do doctors face at the moment?
What is being done to reduce these problems?
Why medicine?
Do you play a lot of sport?
Do you think it's important to diversify to try a lot of new things when you come to university?
Tell me about "Jeans for Genes" (I'd mentioned it on my UCAS form) Do you think genetics is important?
Why medicine?
Why not business?
How do we know if you really mean it, how should we decide who deserves to study medicine or not?
How do you know you want to do medicine?
Any idea what field within medicine you want to do?
What may cause stress in this particular profession?
Tell us about media interests in doctors and the NHS.
What causes you stress?
How would you know if you were stressed?
What have you read recently in the newspapers concerning health/medicine, NOT including MRSA!
Tell me how malaria is controlled.
How does maths help in pursuing a career in the medical profession?

Interview 4
Did you apply to us last year?
What do you think went wrong last year? (no interviews)
Why medicine?
What have you done on your gap year so far?
I see you are doing more work experience. (then he just stared at me so I started to elaborate)
So you think teamwork is important in medicine?
How do you deal with stress?
Let me put you in a stressful situation then. What would you do in a A&E ward if your sister has called you, have a meeting to go to, a

member of staff is missing, a patient needs care immediately……….
etc.
What do you do to relax?
I see you also help at a children's hospice. What do you think of that?
Who is responsible for the children at the hospice? (I still don't totally understand what they meant by this question….)
It must be sad sometimes at the hospice?
What would make you a good doctor)
Why are you learning sign language?
Tell me about a recent medical issue.
What's your opinion on denying treatment to some patients?
Tell me about another medical issue.
What happens once you finish your degree?
What do you think is your biggest weakness?
Do you have any questions about the course at Bristol? (I wish I said nothing on this)
Who have you spoken to about a future medical career?
I didn't understand this on your personal statement. what is a "year 7 sleep over"?
Why are you doing a biology A level this year as well?

Interview 5

Why do you want to be a doctor
Tell us about your work experience
What did you learn from it about the lives of doctors?
What would be the hardest thing, for you, about being a doctor
And what are the other stressful or hard things about being a doctor
How would you cope with these stresses?
How old are you when you become a G.P. or consultant?
Would you be OK with being so old before you fully qualify?
What skills have you learnt in your current work that could transfer to medicine?
Why do you think you have the right personality for medicine?
What have you read about in terms of medical research or the NHS that has interested you? What issues does it raise?

Cambridge: St Catherine's

Two consecutive interviews of about 25 min. each with dean and pre-clinical medicine director of studies
General interview with dean

Why medicine?
Are you sure, thought about anything else?
Have I completed Duke of Edinburgh, what left to do, bit about tae kwon do and other activities on personal statement.
Have you worked with elderly/experienced dirtier and less attractive aspects of medicine?
What would you do if as a junior doctor you gave someone 10 times as much of a drug as you were supposed to?
And your career?
Some factual, AS knowledge questions about the heart and how carbon dioxide is transport in the blood, quite specific.
About buffers in the body
Subject interview with DoS
If you were washed up on a desert island, what medicines would you want washed up with you?
What do you think are the priorities for improving health in the 3rd world?
What is the human genome?
How many genes in the human genome?
Why do rice plants have several times more genes than humans?
Name some genetic diseases.
Tell me about cystic fibrosis.
Tell me about Huntington's disease.
What do you think about testing for late onset diseases?
Tell me about a piece of research that has interested you recently.
Name an invention in the 18th? Century that has revolutionised the way that we think about disease (microscope)
Why don't you think that we have made very fast progress in producing a vaccine against malaria?
Why have imaging devices been so useful?

Any questions?
It doesn't worry you that this is a very science based course?

Cambridge St John's College:,

Background

BMAT sat on November 1st. Results back at end of month (Got score of 26). No further tests, and no mention of BMAT results in interview. No work requested. Interviews all in a single day. Given free meal, no accommodation.

Interviews
Two interviews:
General interview, specifically on personal statement. With admissions tutor in charge of medicine (who happened to be the Dean) and a medical professional (apparently, usually head of the clinical course at St John's, but just a doctor this time). Friendly atmosphere, comfy room. Genuinely felt they had read personal statement very closely and that this was a considered interview.
Questions included:
Describe how science is taught at your school. What teaching styles are you exposed to?
Your class sizes are quite large. How does this affect you?
What do you particularly like about your school?
Were you coached on the BMAT at all?
Why Drama at AS level?
Do you think there are any skills you can bring from this to medicine?
What is this Murder Mystery business? What is a murder mystery? Relates to medicine how?
What hospital work experience did you do? Learnt what?
If you saw someone cheating in a BMAT exam, what would you do?
If this person went on to become a doctor, and he had a drinking
If you saw someone cheating in a BMAT exam, what would you do?
If this person went on to become a doctor, and he had a drinking

problem, would you feel obliged to tell your superiors? Would you feel guilty that he became a doctor because you didn't speak up? Any questions?

Medical / scientific interview.
With head of pre-clinical at St John's and University wide pathology professor. Again, very light and friendly. Comfy room, full of skeletons and models, pictures and sofas. Questioning was probing, but they were very helpful and guided you through problems.
Define science.
Describe the causes of cancer.
Why does a particular carcinogen cause cancer in the bladder but nowhere else?

At this point, they went on a highly amusing sojourn into eulogising about how my personal statement was a nice change they liked the self deprecation apparently. And then started quoting sections at me ("getting thrashed by Alzheimer's patients at dominoes"), and debating whether their condition would affect their ability to give me a good whipping at board games. I was thoroughly baffled at this point. But eventually, we got back to questions.

What observations are taken in a hospital?
How is blood pressure measured?

Interview 2

Two 35 minute interviews. Panel of 2 each time (one medical fellow and one practising clinician)
 Much harder. Much more science based. Talked a bit about ethics of 22 week resuscitation and about drug trials. But mainly science. They prompted a lot. Had to think very hard as you can't learn what they will ask. They were more challenging than the Bristol ones. Also, they wanted to see if you were confident with your answers "are you sure?" Which made me doubt my answers and change them even if they were initially right.

Cardiff University School of Medicine

Why I wanted to be a doctor,
What were the difficulties,
Things about my work experience,
What makes a good team,
What areas of medicine my volunteering things would be helpful with,
Why Cardiff.

Glasgow

Interview 1

Why medicine?
What have I been doing since I left school (as I am a graduate)
What do I think of PBL
Why not social work (as I have a lot of care experience)
Why do other faculties/university's not use PBL
What is medical issues have I seen in the news

Dundee, University of, Faculty of Medicine, Dentistry and Nursing

Interview 1
Interview was 15 mins with 2 people. very relaxed.
Asked me why I wanted to be a doctor
Question about the pressures on doctors
Medicine is a profession, what does this entail,?
What are the drawbacks of it
What current medical issue in the news,
Why do you want to come to Dundee
What happens between the time a pharmacist invents a drug and a doctor prescribing it.

Interview 2

There are several interviews going on at once in the same room, I was interviewed by two people, I think one was a medic and one was a medic/academic. They were both really nice and the interview was very relaxed and informal. I think it lasted about 15 minutes. I was mainly asked questions relating to my personal statement, but as I am a graduate applicant this may not be the standard format also the other applicants who I spoke to afterwards had all been asked different questions so I guess it all depends on which pair of interviewers you get assigned to. There were about 40 applicants there when I went half get a tour of the medical school while the other half are interviewed. I reckon it's better to do the tour first, because then you probably have more to talk about

Durham, University of, Queens Campus, Stockton, Phase I Medicine

East Anglia, University of

Interview 1
What have you done on your gap year?
Experience of being a Doctor
Example of Teamwork? What would you do if a member of your team was slacking?
What is your greatest achievement non academically and academically?
Why should we give you the offer and not the others?
Something that I've found challenging in my work experience?

Interview 2
I attended an interview on the 17th of January at the University of East Anglia. A group of 7 candidates, including myself, went in to the interview room. There were seven "stations" around the room, each with one interviewer. All of us candidates had to rotate separately around the seven stations. There was a time limit of five minutes per station and we were asked around 4 questions.

Each station had a theme on which the questions would be based. The themes are as follows;
1) Teamwork
2) Ethical Scenario 1 involving a patient
3) Ethical Scenario 2 involving a colleague/close friend
4) About the course at University of East Anglia
5) Something you have done that you are proud of
6) What sets you apart from other candidates and what genre of medicine you are interested in
7) Time management

Edinburgh, The University of, The Faculty of Medicine

Interview 1
There are two panels, one with two guys and one with two lovely older women!

No ethics questions or anything on the health care system
Why medicine and why Edinburgh?
For graduates why now and not when you left school
Questioned about work experience
Explain your strengths and weaknesses
What advise would I give freshers
Name a book you have read recently which has influenced your life and how?
The main body of questions were follow on from any answer I gave to the above,

Interview 2
Why now and not before,
Why Edinburgh
Asked if I was wanting to be a clinical academic.
How I would fit in with the younger ones.
Was given a sheet to read before the interview with BMJ editorials?
Was not asked about them in the end

Apart from why Edinburgh, why now
I did get asked to summarise one of the editorials we were given at the start! It was something about children with depression and what not to treat them with.
He then asked me how I would diagnose a patient with depression not just whether they were sad or something.

I had two guys interviewing me as well and got the journals on depression and dignity in medicine but almost all my interview was on ethics, it was a bit of a nightmare and they went through my CV to check if I was lying about hobbies.
Also I told them that I did not do Biology at school because it was mainly plant biology to which they answered why don't plants have brains!
However, my interview was only 20 mins long even though it was supposed to be 45 mins.

I was asked quite a lot about euthanasia and what I would do and if I thought the law should be changed and how it was different to suicide. They also asked me about cloning

Interview 3
Why medicine?,
Why now, and the rest was about my personal statement.
"So I see you got an essay prize in your second year at university for an essay on the Chandra telescope…"
"Yes, I did, but I didn't realise I'd written that on my ps, it doesn't really have anything to do with wanting to be a doctor"
"So can you tell me a bit about the Chandra telescope?"
Another priceless moment was when I mentioned that I was interested in immunology with respect to going into transplant surgery.
"Surgery, oh, you know you have to be pretty good with your hands to do that. Do you do any practical things with your hands, like drawing, painting, or cooking, something like that?
"Yes, actually, in my final year at school I studied a tailoring course

in my spare time, and now I design and make shirts."
Then... "So, I was just wondering, do you make wall hangings, and things like that "
"Eh?" :shock:
"I mean like little things you can hang on the wall or mantelpiece" (laugh) " I can't believe we're having this conversation, are you looking for something specific? I've never tried to do curtains"
"Well, I was just wondering if it was the human body that you liked making things for."

So, advice for anyone who still has theirs to go... Make sure you try and steer the conversation onto your love for medicine, and everything they ask you, should try and put a medical slant on it (And when they ask you things like "So, do you read much?" I think you should probably answer with a medical book.

Hull York Medical School

HYMS send a list of potential questions, prepare using these. Interviewed January outcome within 2 weeks

Admissions
Potential interview questions for admission to HYMS
We interview applicants in order to get to know you better as a person, to try to assess how your attitudes, creativity and personality will contribute to you as a doctor There are no 'right answers' to the interview questions. The interviewers are genuinely interested in your expression of your personal opinions and feelings, your discussion of your own experiences and your ability to explore issues from a number of different viewpoints.
This sample list of questions gives you an idea of the topic areas and the sorts of questions you may be asked. We will be using similar, but not necessarily the same, questions as shown here, so do not try to learn answers to the questions listed. You will do best in your interview if you listen carefully and then try to answer the question you are asked, rather than if you give a prepared answer. Candidates

who appear over coached put themselves at a disadvantage.

Knowledge of Problem Based Learning and the Hull York Medical School (HYMS)

To explore how well you will thrive in the particular learning environment provided by the Hull York Medical School. An appreciation of PBL is essential.

1. What appeals to you or interests you about the course here at HYMS?
2. What previous experiences have you had of learning in a small group setting?
3. What do you know about the course at the Hull York Medical School? How did you find this out?
4. Tell us what attracts you most and least about the Hull and York Medical School.
5. What do you know about PBL? Why do you want to come to a PBL medical school?
6. What do you think are the advantages and disadvantages of a PBL course? Why do you think it will suit you personally?
7. What do you think are the advantages and disadvantages of coming to a new medical school?
8. This course will require a good deal of independent study, how have you managed this approach to learning in the past?
9. How did you first find out about HYMS? What do you know about PBL? Why do you think PBL will suit you personally?

Motivation for medicine

To explore the driving forces behind your personal desire to be a doctor, and your awareness of your own strengths and weaknesses.

10. Why do you want to be a doctor
11. What do you want to achieve in medicine? How do you see your career in ten years time?
12. What have you read or experienced in order to prepare you for medicine?
13. Why do you believe you have the ability to undertake the study and work involved?
14. Why do you want to be a doctor, rather than another profession

that is caring or intellectually challenging?
15. What do you think the job of being a doctor entails, other than treating patients? Will this suit you?
16. When you think about becoming a doctor, what do you look forward to most and least?
17. What impact do you hope to make in the field of medicine?
18. Why study medicine rather than any other health care profession? How do you think the role of doctors differs from other health professions, such as specialist nurse practitioners?
19. What aspect of health care attracts you to medicine?
20. Why do you want to be a doctor What steps have you taken to find out whether this is really right for you?
21. There are many different ways of helping people. Why do you want to study medicine, rather than working in any other health or social care professions?
22. Can you tell us about any particular life experiences that you think may help or hinder you in a career in medicine?

Depth and breadth of interest
To explore how you have read, researched and reflected about medicine and about the wider world.
23. Can you tell us about a significant recent advance in medicine or science? Why is it significant? Why has this interested you?
24. What do you consider to be important advance in medicine over the last 50 / 100 years?
25. Can you tell us about a significant medical story in the media at the moment? [Supp: What do you think are the key issues here?]
26. Tell us about something in the history of medicine that interests you. Why was it important?
27. Tell us about a film or book that has influenced you or made you think recently, and why?
28. What do you think is the most important medical discovery in the last 100 200 years, and why?
29. If a benefactor offered you a huge amount of money to set up a Medical Research Institute and invited you to become its director, what research area would you choose to look at, and why?
30. Tell us about someone who has been a major influence on you as

a person / in your life?

31. What do you think was the greatest public health advance of the twentieth century?

32. Can you describe an interesting place you have been to (need not be medical or exotic) and explain why it was so?

33. Do you think putting a man on the moon money well spent? If yes why? If no how would you have spent that money?

34. How do you think the rise in information technology has influenced / will influence the practice of medicine?

Work Experience

To explore how you respond to, and reflect on, the emotional and practical challenges experienced in a work environment

35. What steps have you taken to find out whether medicine is really the right career for you?

36. What experiences have given you insight into the world of medicine? What have you learnt from these?

37. What aspect of your work experience did you find the most challenging, and why?

38. Through your work experience, what skills have you learnt that you can apply to medicine?

39. Thinking of your work experience, can you tell me about a difficult situation you have dealt with and what you learned from it?

40. Have you visited any friends or family in hospital, or had work experience in a hospital? From these experiences, what did you see that you would like to change, and why?

41. Can you tell me the key things you learned from your work experience, in caring or other settings?

42. What have you done on work experience / in employment previously? What would you change about what you saw, if you could, and how would you set about this?

43. Tell me about a project, or work experience, that you have organised, and what you learned from it?

44. Describe briefly one situation in which you have had work experience. What were the best and worse features? How could you change them?

Team work

To explore your experience and understanding of the challenges and problems of working in a team

45. Thinking about your membership of a team (in a work, sport, school or other setting), can you tell us about the most important contributions you made to the team?

46. Think of a team situation where your communication skills have been vital. Tell us about the situation and your contribution.

47. Tell us about a group activity you have organised. What went well and what went badly? What did you learn from it?

48. Can you give me an example of how you coped with a conflict with a colleague or friend; what strategy did you use and why?

49. Tell us about a team situation you have experienced. What did you learn about yourself and about successful team working?

50. When you think about yourself working as a doctor, who do you think will be the most important people that you will be working with?

51. Who do you think are the important members of a multi disciplinary health care team? Why?

52. What are the advantages and disadvantages of being in a team? How can you help a team to develop?

53. Can you give examples of teams with and without leaders? Do health care teams need leaders? Why/ why not?

54. Modern day health care is very much a team effort. Please tell us a role that you have played in a team, and what you think you contributed.

55. What do you think are the advantages and disadvantages of nurses replacing doctors as the first contact person in the primary care team?

Personal Insight

To explore your assessment of your strengths and weaknesses and how you think you can to build on both of these.

56. What ways of working and studying have you developed that you think will assist you through medical school? What will you need to improve?

57. There is a great deal to be covered in the medical curriculum, but nevertheless students at HYMS have a half day free on Wednesdays

for sport. Do you think we should we incorporate Wednesday afternoons into the medical timetable?

58. Medical training is long and being a doctor can be stressful. Some doctors who qualify never practice. What makes you think you will stick to it?

59. What do you think will be the most difficult things you might encounter during your training? How will you deal with them?

60. Is there such a thing as positive criticism? How do you think you will cope with criticism from colleagues or other health professionals?

61. Why do you think doctors nowadays sued much more often than, say, twenty years ago? How do you think you would cope with being criticised or even sued?

62. Give us an example of something about which you used to hold strong opinions, but have had to change your mind. What made you change? What do you think now?

63. Have you ever been in a situation where you realise afterwards that what you said or did was wrong? What did you do about it? What should you have done?

64. What are your outside interests and hobbies? How do these compliment you as a person? Which do you think you will continue at university?

65. How do you think you personally will judge whether you have been successful in your life? What aspects of your life will you consider?

66. What relevance to medicine are the 'A' levels (apart from biology and chemistry) that you have been studying?

67. What do you think the phrase 'work life balance' means? Why could it be difficult for you to achieve?

68. What do you think you will be the positive aspects and the negative aspects of being a doctor How will you handle these?

69. Can you tell us about an interesting experience, and what you learned from it about yourself?

70. What qualities do you think other people value in you? What characteristics do you think you would most need to change in the course of becoming a good doctor

71. What do you think are your priorities in your own personal

development?

72. Tell me three words that you think your friends would use to describe you. What personal qualities do you need to improve to become a good doctor

Understanding of the role of medicine in society

To explore your thoughts and understanding of how medical care fits in with how society is organised

73. Medicine is often said to be both an art and a science. Which aspects do you think are art and which are science?
74. How do politics influence health care provision? Is it inevitable?
75. What do you think of nurses developing extended roles and undertaking tasks previously done by doctors?
76. In what ways do you think doctors can promote good health, other than direct treatment of illness?
77. From what you have read and found out, where do you see the health service going?
78. What are the arguments for and against nonessential surgery being available on the NHS?
79. Why do you think an NHS Trust has recently proposed to limit the access of very obese patients to certain types of surgery? [Supp: Can you think of any arguments for / against this?]
80. What does the current government see as the national priorities in health care? Do you agree with these?
81. What do you think are the similarities and differences between being a doctor today and being a doctor 50 years ago?
82. Should doctors have a role in regulating contact sports, such as boxing?
83. Do you think doctors should ever go on strike?
84. Do you think patient's treatments should be limited by the NHS budget or do they have the right to new therapies no matter what the cost?
85. What does the term 'inequalities in health' mean to you?
86. What do you think is the purpose of the health service in the 21st century?
87. Why do you think people in the north of England live, on average, 5 years less than those in the south? Do you think this

should be a matter for government intervention?
88. What are the arguments for and against people paying for their own health care as and when they need it?
89. Where do you think the bulk of medical treatment takes place: hospital or in the community? What makes you think this?
90. What do you think about the way doctors are shown in the media, say in the Simpsons or on the news? How do you think this will affect patients' views of their own doctors?
91. What do you think is the greatest threat to the health of the British population today?
92. What do you think will be the key tasks of doctors in 40 years time?
93. Ten years ago most doctors in hospitals wore white coats; now few do. Why do you think this is? What do you think are the arguments for and against white coats?
94. Do you think more doctors or more nurses would be of greatest benefit to the nation's health?
95. What are the arguments for and against banning the sale of tobacco?
96. In the UK at present 60% of medical students are female. Do you think we should have equal quotas for medical school places for males and females? What do you think are the consequences of having more doctors of one sex than the other?
97. What problems do you think the widespread use of recreational drugs pose to doctors?
98. What issues should be considered in deciding to terminate or not continue a patient's life sustaining treatment?
99. Was it right that George Best had a liver transplant? [Supp: explore reasons for or against}
100. Medicine will bring you into contact with a vast range of different people, with different cultures; what experience have you had of different types of people?
Tolerance of uncertainty
To explore how you try to make a rational decision in the face of incomplete or conflicting information or when the outcome has different consequences for different people.

101. Is it better to give health care or aid to impoverished countries? What do you think about the activities of charities such as Medecins sans Frontiers?

102. What do you think would be the advantages, and difficulties, for a person with a major physical disability (e.g. blindness) wishing to become a doctor

103. What reasons are there for involving patients in medical decision making?

104. Do you think we should find out more about patients' views of their doctors, their illness or their treatments? How would you set about this?

105. What do you think are the major sorts of problems facing a person with a long-term health problem, such as difficulty breathing? How can a doctor help?

106. Should a doctor be able to claim 'conscientious objection' from providing a medical treatment?

107. Why do you think it is that we cannot give a guarantee that a medical or surgical procedure will be successful?

108. Imagine you are on committee able to recommend only one of two new surgical treatments to be made available through the NHS. The treatments are: an artificial heart for babies born with heart defects, or a permanent replacement hip for people with severe arthritis. Both treatments are permanent, i.e. never need repeating, and are of equal cost. On what grounds would you make your arguments?

109. Should alternative or complimentary medicine be funded by the NHS, and why / why not?

110. How do you think doctors should treat injury or illness due to self harm, smoking or excess alcohol consumption?

111. Female infertility treatment is expensive, has a very low success rate and is even less successful in smokers. To whom do you think it should be available?

112. How do you respond and what do you feel when you see a beggar in the street?

113. You have one liver available for transplant, but two patients with equal medical need. One is an ex alcoholic mother with

two young children, the other a 13 year old with an inborn liver abnormality. How would you decide to whom it should be given?
114. What do you think about the use of animals for testing new drugs?

Imperial

Typical questions include;

Concerning motivation and a realistic approach to medicine as a career:
What have you done to find out about medicine as a career. Who have you talked to about doing medicine and what did you learn from them?
What do you think you might like best about medicine as a career?
What do you feel are likely to be the worst things about being a doctor
When you visited a hospital, what did you see that set you thinking about the difficult aspects of a medical career?
What skills do you have that would make you a good doctor
What do you feel makes a good doctor
What difference did your work experience make to you?
Response to stress:
What do you do to relax?
How do you cope in situations where there is not enough time to finish a task?
We all know exams are stressful. How did you manage when you were taking your GCSEs?
What do you do when you have 3 or 4 things to do that are all urgent?
Evidence of working both as a leader and team member; ability to multi task:
Have you dealt with a difficult situation?
I see you are captain of a team. What duties does that involve?
How do you feel about sharing work with others?
How do you balance work and all your outside activities?

I see you play sport/do the Duke of Ed/play in the orchestra (or similar) Why is this important to you?
I see you were Director/Manager in your Young Enterprise company. How did you go about performing this role?
Contribution to Medical School life:
Which activities do you think you would like to do?
Would you like to do something new or continue your music/drama/mountaineering (or similar)?
What would you like people to remember about you from your medical school life?
The medical course is hard work. How do you propose to manage your work and still play football/violin (or similar)?

Interview 1
Why do you want to be a doctor If you couldn't do medicine what would you do? Would you like to be a nurse?
What qualities do a doctor need? Do you think a doctor's job is stressful? How do you deal with stress?
A banker works long hours – why is he different from a doctor
What do you do to relax? Do you read?
Sell yourself to us for 2 minutes.
Are you a people person or a loner? Do you enjoy working in a team?
Tell me about a situation where you have shown leadership skills.
Have you ever experienced death?
Does anyone in your family work in the medical profession?
Have you ever considered taking a gap year?
In ten years time after you have become a doctor and all your friends wants to have a reunion but you are unable to attend, so how would you want them to remember you?
I see you come from a different country, what is it like there?
How can you relate being a doctor to the piano?

Interview 2
What contribution could you make to this medical school? What outside activities would you be prepared to do here? What extra curricular activities would you like to get involved in if you came

here?
Why do you want to come to Imperial?
How did you prepare for this interview?
How do you think the Systems and Topics based course going to help the future of medicine?
Explain your choices of university. Why did you choose 3 London medical schools and Nottingham? If you like the systems based course, why did you apply to Cambridge?
Tell us about your work experience. What did you learn from it?
Do you remember any particular patients that didn't have a good outcome? Did you see any patients that had a good outcome?
What have you done to find out about the career? (Discussed work experience why do you like it? What has it taught you?)
What kind of voluntary work did you do?
You seem to have a wide variety of work experience but seem to lack work experience at a G.P.'s practice and in hospital. Have you done anything that you have not mentioned?
What was your House Officer like where you went for WE?
Has a patient you've been close to ever died? Do you feel that you would feel emotion?

Interview 3
What do you think most people who qualify in medicine do? (over 50% become G.P.s)
Have you ever considered becoming a G.P.?
Why do you think the suicide rate in doctors is so high? What would stop you committing suicide as a doctor
Did you know your local health authority has the largest number of bed blockers? How should the NHS go about removing bed blockers?
What is wrong with the NHS?
What is Down's syndrome? Can you describe a down's syndrome child?
Tell us about any medical articles you have seen in the media recently.
What announcements has Alan Milburn made recently?

(Referring to my personal statement) What are your opinions on alternative medicines?
Who do you think should be leaders in the field of medicine?
Are there any advantages/disadvantages to the "human Genome Project"? What sort of laws should be passed on to prevent people taking advantages over this?
You said that you were interested in cloning, what do you think of stem cell research and the possibility of using it to treat diabetes?
What if you made a mistake while giving a patient his regular dosage, what would you do?
What if you had a patient with an incurable disease, what can you do about it?
You said that the patient you described had diabetes and therefore was not a candidate for renal transplant, do you think that is fair? As I have a patient that has a diabetes and has just received a transplant?

Interview 4
Do you know what the NHS Plan is?
Tell me about your job at the Cromwell Hospital.
What do you look forward to most about coming to medical school?
I see that your father is a doctor, what type of doctor is he?
Has he influenced you in any way to become a doctor
What do you think patients see as the good qualities in a doctor
Would you empathise or sympathise?
If you had the blood test of some one who was terminally ill and they came through your door, what would you say?
If they are terminally ill, there is nothing we can do, should we just leave them alone?
Would you say that I have failed if one of my patients dies on me?
So you say you like cricket and that you attend cricket matches, what started your interest?
What do you believe will happen in the England Vs India series?
What do you believe has been the biggest recent breakthrough in medicine recently?
What else affects heart disease?
I read that you went on the Medlink course, what in particular did

this teach you about medicine?
If I gave you £100,000 to go to a third world countries, how would you use it?
What other diseases are there in third world countries?
Where are cholera and typhoid found?
How do you intend to spend your gap year and why?

Interview 5

What sort of doctor would I like to be?
What is the relevance of sciences to the study of medicine?
What do you think about imperial as a university?
More questions about my hobbies and interests.....
What was the last book/article I read about medicine?
Where do I intend to practice medicine after graduation (watch out if you are an overseas student!)
What did you learn from your work experience
How would you cope in telling a patient relative that the patient died
Why do you want to do surgery ultimately
Why medicine
How will you contribute to the university
Give examples of where you have used teamwork and leadership skills
If you were the prime minister what 3 government policies would you set to achieve?
What's more important caring or intellect?
What did you do for Duke of Edinburgh?
What's the best thing you saw in your work experience at G.P.?
Have you ever been a leader?
Have you ever had to make an unpopular decision as a leader?
Do you prefer to be a leader or a member of a team?
How would you contribute to imperial college?
How do you de-stress?
What will you do if a patient turns aggressive towards you?

Interview 6
Everyone got a case study of some sort/question, and were meant to discuss it for a few minutes, I got 'should all fertility treatment be treated on the NHS?' I went in with the pros and cons
What are the disadvantages of choosing gametes/embryos etc
And the regular questions: why imperial
What are the good qualities of a doctor
What demonstrates your teamwork skills?
What demonstrates your leadership skills?
What could you offer to imperial?
You say that you read the Independent, what have you read from it?
After I talked about a medical research. I'm a neurologist why do you think it's difficult to develop a vaccine for that
You say that you're scrupulous/moral what do you mean by that ..?
What was your work experience like /how did you get it?
Then they said we will let you know in two weeks/any questions?

Interview 7
You're from Wales, why have you chosen to come all the way here to London to study?
Have you had a chance to look around our campus?
What first inspired you to become a doctor
What did you learn from your work experience?
You read the newspapers I presume Could you please tell me of a recent article that caught your eye.
What are the biggest challenges that face doctors today?
What's the difference between the French health system and ours? (related to my work experience in a French clinic.)
You're a partner in a G.P. surgery, a new person comes in to register for the first time, what questions do you ask and what tests do you carry out?
 What sports teams would you join if you came here? (the medical students always ask the nice ones!)
Any questions?

Interview 8

The Totally Brilliant Medicourses Interview Book

How do you deal with stress?
Was doing gold Duke of Edinburgh worth it? Assorted questions about group organisation during the expedition etc
What do you think most doctors do?
What speciality do you see yourself following?
Not a G.P.? Why not?
Why did you find radiology so interesting?

Talked about the case study for 2 mins "should a smoker be given a lung transplant on the NHS"
What do you think makes a good doctor
What stood out for you in your work experience.
You seem to be achieving v.high grades....why??
Have you ever failed? How did that make you feel?
If somebody on your team made a mistake, what would you do?
If you made a mistake with a patient, what would you do?
What can you offer to Imperial
Why Imperial?

Interview 9
You should have been given a question, "Should a doctor be allowed to prescribe contraception to an underage patient without the knowledge of the parents?", What are your thoughts on this?
I see you take part in a lot of activities at school and outside of school. How have these given you experience in working in a team?
How do doctors work as teams? And why is their cooperation important?
If you had an uncooperative member of your team what would you do to get them more involved.
I see you like football, has that given you any experience of being in a position of leadership?
Oh yes, I meant to check this out but didn't have time, your web site, what is that all about?
I see you have taken part in the Nuffield bursary scheme at GSK.. What did that entail?
So what make you want to become a doctor instead of a boffin

researcher?
Have you heard of another viruses that may be featuring in the news recently?
Yes, so how do viruses 'jump species'?
And so how does that effect vaccinations?
Well, for instance why do scientists find it so hard to make a flu vaccination?
Out of all the things you do what do you find the most enjoyable?
Do you have a favourite author?

Interview 10
How are you?
Where have you come from?
How did you get here?
So you have your 4 A's already, is that right?
What have you been doing recently?
You say in your personal statement that drama helped you with your communication skills. How did it do this?
Beyond this, the order of the questions is all blurred, but here are the questions I remember:
What are the qualities in a good doctor
Do you know what NICE is? Tell me about what it does.
What's wrong with NICE?
Do you think that drugs should be introduced quicker than they are? (They went on to a discussion about herceptin)
Why is it important for there to be a balance between work and outside of work activities?
Other than academically, how would you contribute to Imperial?
What is the difference between the job of a nurse and a doctor
Do you think it's OK for nurses to be given some of the responsibilities of doctors?
What is the ethos of medicine?
Do you have any disabilities you want to tell us about?
Do you have any questions for us?
I assume you read a broadsheet newspaper? What recent piece of medical news have you read?

Interview 11
Do you think that drugs should reach the market faster?
Do you think NICE is as efficient as they should be?
Do you know what NICE actually do?
So why medicine?
When was it when you realised you wanted to do medicine?
So you said on your personal statement you are looking for more work experience have you arranged any more?
What was the most memorable thing about your work experience in A&E when you were 16?
What was the last medical article you read?
You also said your looking for a job, have you got one?
You mention a lot about kung fu what has this done for you?
How important do you think it is too keep a balance of work and hobbies?
Any questions?

Interview 12
Have you seen the college?
How would you encourage people to donate organs?
How about in schools?
Do you have any experience in dealing with patients? Who influenced you to apply for medicine?
Reference to personal statement: It seems that you are sometimes unsure if you want to do medicine?
Apart from music, what do you think you can contribute to Imperial?
What books have you read? How do you think these help prepare you for medical school?

Imperial medical School base their interview marking on the following criteria.
Leadership
Team working
Ethical question

Work experience
Contribution to the medical School

Keele, University of, School of Medicine

Each interview lasts 20 minutes (no more, no less). The interview panel comprises 3 interviewers and a chairman. The majority of the interviewers are practising clinicians. The candidate will not have the opportunity to ask questions of the interviewers or chairman. Any questions that candidate may have can be raised during the remainder of the day.

The interview is not a test of candidates' academic knowledge. Candidates will not be asked questions directly related to their curriculum. The pre-interview screening process operated by the School of Medicine (based on academic grading, personal statement and school/college reference) will already have assured that all candidates called to interview are of sufficient academic calibre. The purpose of the interview is to assess the candidate as a whole person.

The interviewers will expect the candidates to be nervous and will of course make allowances for this. In most cases, outward signs of nervousness evaporate within two or three minutes of starting the interview.

The interview panel, in addition to forming an overall impression of the student, will be assessing in particular the following areas:

1. Ability to communicate. Communication skills are essential to the practice of almost all aspects of medicine. We expect candidates to be able to express their ideas clearly and coherently and to be able to follow a reasoned argument. Candidates who give spontaneous yet well thought out answers to questions are more likely to impress the interviewers than those who give obviously rehearsed and "coached" responses. There are clearly some questions which schools and students will anticipate (see below) but during the course of the

interview there will be other questions which occur spontaneously to the interviewers and cannot be anticipated by the students.

2. Why does candidate wish to be a doctor This is an obvious though vital question. It is also the question to which candidates most frequently reply with a coached and practised answer. This is not to say that practised answers would entirely rule a candidate out of consideration, however they are clearly not as impressive as answers which are spontaneous and show genuine flair and enthusiasm for the subject.

3. Does the student have genuine outside interests? Candidates can expect to be asked at some length about their hobbies and interests, and other non academic pursuits. Obviously a starting point for these questions will be areas the candidate has mentioned on his/her personal statement. Clearly, this may lead onto other areas but candidates should be aware that anything they write on their personal statement is "fair game" for question at interview. Thus candidates are advised to be careful when compiling their personal statement and not to include a list of "hobbies" with which they have only a passing interest, merely to compile a list.

Interviewers themselves have a wide range of interests, which often include many of those cited by candidates! The panel is not at all concerned as to exactly what candidates outside interests are merely to assess whether they are able to talk about them with some degree of knowledge and enthusiasm.

4. Previous caring experience. Any experience of a caring role will clearly be a topic raised by the interviewers. This role need not be in a medical environment. The interview is an opportunity for candidates to relate not only the facts and details of their role but also their emotional response to it, what it has taught them, and what they have gained from it.

5. Matters of a "medical interest". Candidates will not be expected to

have knowledge of details of medical processes. However, the panel will feel it reasonable to expect the candidate to have an intelligent lay person's view on many aspects of medicine particularly those of current media interest. Ethical problem may be raised for discussion but candidates should be reassured that neither the panel nor the School of Medicine will take a position on any ethical issue. It is not the candidate's ethical views that the panel may be interested in but how coherently the candidate expresses those views.

6. Candidates may be asked about different problems or situations as part of the interview that may or may not include those of a medical nature. Candidates will not require any specialist knowledge for this section of the interview. The purpose is to test "thought processes" rather than knowledge.

Interview 1
Keele University interview
Why do you want to be a doctor
Why don't you want to be a nurse as they have quite similar roles?
Why keele university?
Why have you chosen to do a PBL course?
What do you think this will involve?
How would you like to be remembered by your fellow students?
What qualities would you bring to the university?
What would you do if you found out your friend was having problems while at university which is affecting her work?

I was also given a current ethical issue where I had to explain my feelings
Toward and debate this with the interviewers. Mine was the MMR triple
vaccine, although I know that one of the issues from this years interviews
is obesity.

King's College London School of Medicine (at Guy's, King's

College and St Thomas' Hospitals)

Interview 1
Candidate given a questionnaire to complete prior to interview;

Why do you want to study medicine?
Why do you want to study at Kings?
Which non science subject you are or have studied, do you feel contributes most to medicine and why?
What qualities make a good or bad doctor
What are the negative and positive aspects in a doctor's career?
What can you contribute to medical School

Prior to interview, also given a dilemma; 'there is a new drug released, it is beneficial to a patients condition. The patient goes to his G.P. who refuses to prescribe the drug; discuss the moral and ethical considerations
What are you covering in each of your subjects recently
How would you handle an aggressive patient?
Do you feel the human genome project is the answer to the medical dilemma?
What do you feel about nurses being able to prescribe drugs?
Discussion of G.P.s rationing drugs
Do you know the name of an expensive drug?
What is the difference between nurses and doctors?
What does NICE do?
Questioned on personal statement, languages and sports

Interview 2

What sparked your interest in a career in medicine?
How did you make sure this was the right career for you?
You said you read the student BMJ, what have you read recently that interested you?
If you had a large sum of money to spend on improving Britain's health care system, what aspect would you spend it on?

How do you deal with pressure? Give an example of a situation where you have had to deal with pressure.
Have you done something challenging recently? What?
Why have you applied to study medicine at this university?
What work experience have you done? Who organised it?
What did you gain from your work experience?
What do you do for fun?

Interview 3

Why do you want to do medicine?
What did you learn about the routine on doctors in your work experience?
Was your work experience beneficial?
What have you learnt from Tae KwonDo that will help you as a doctor
What did you learn from your trip to Pfizer?
What is the atmosphere like in a hospice? What type of care do they provide?
Do you believe this atmosphere contributes to the public's view of doctors being arrogant?
Case study about patient going to his/her G.P. with information of internet telling them about a better drug then the one they are being prescribed. What issues does the G.P. face?
Is the internet a good thing for patients? How is it dangerous

Interview 4

Pre-interview
Fill in questionnaire beforehand. Simple questions like:
Why medicine?
Why King's?
Have you done anything recently that you are particularly proud of?
How have you shown you are responsible and trustworthy?
What work experience have you completed?
This questionnaire is meant to be taken into the interview and

looked at by the interviewers. They didn't actually look at mine until after the interview.

You are also given an ethical scenario to look over. 20 minutes given for both of these… I found it quite rushed.

The Interview

The interview itself was quite friendly, more of a discussion than an intense grilling. The interview panel was two consultants, one of whom took control of part 1, the other part 2, although both contributed to each. The interview room was basically a few armchairs and a small table. It lasted about 15 minutes.

Interview 5

Part 1: Questions on Personal Statement and General Medical Issues
Why medicine?
Why at King's?
Describe some of your hospital work experience and what you learnt from it
The future of the NHS… dealing with payment by results, choose and book, the new IT system, F1s and F2s.
What are the advantages / disadvantages of this system?
You say you like reading… describe a book you've read recently.

Part 2: Ethical Scenario
Similar to ethical scenario on bottom of p95 of A Very Short Introduction to Medical Ethics by Tony Hope.
Prompted to discuss issues… e.g.: Abortion
Confidentiality (particularly: is genetic information solely an individuals or should it be shared family wide?"
Sanctity of life
Received response via UCAS within two weeks.

Interview 6

What makes a good doctor What skills should they have?

What have you read in the BMJ / The New scientist recently that has really interested you?
What did you learn from your work experience?
What surprised you on you work experience at the hospital?

I was given an ethical dilemma and questioned about it. I had to imagine I was a junior doctor and my senior doctor had just been widowed but continued working and because of this was making some errors at work. I was asked what would I do.

Leicester, University of, School of Medicine

Liverpool, University of, Faculty of Medicine

What was PBL,
What is an integrated course
What did I think of running an integrated course
How would I cope with the pressures of being a medical student/doctor
Give an example of when I had shown initiative
How have I got time management skills
How have I got leadership/ teamwork skills,
Have I done any reading about medicine.

Manchester, University of, Faculty of Medicine, Dentistry, Pharmacy and Nursing

Short listed candidates will be called for interview in the Medical school. No candidate will be offered a place at Manchester without an interview. Occasionally, applicants arrive for interview even when they are feeling unwell. If you are not feeling 100%, please tell the admissions staff before the interview; we will be happy to reschedule it. Please understand that we cannot accept pleas of infirmity after the interview.

The interview itself is a formal though friendly process. Each interview lasts 15 minutes. The interview panel comprises three (occasionally two) interviewers and a chairperson. The majority of the interviewers are practising clinicians. The candidate will not have the opportunity to ask questions of the interviewers or chairman. Any questions that the candidate may have can be raised during the remainder of the day.

The interview is not a test of a candidate's academic knowledge. The pre-interview screening process operated by the Medical School (based on academic grading, personal statement and reference) will already have ensured that all candidates called to interview appear to have sufficient academic potential. The purpose of the interview is to take a wider view of the applicant as described below.

The interviewers appreciate that some candidates will be nervous and will of course make allowances for this. In most cases, outward signs of nervousness evaporate within two or three minutes of starting the interview. We do try to be friendly but are aware that we can be perceived as threatening. That is certainly not our intention.

Ability to communicate

Communication skills are essential to the practice of almost all aspects of medicine. We expect candidates to be able to express their ideas clearly and coherently and to be able to follow a reasoned argument. Candidates who give spontaneous yet well thought out answers to questions are more likely to impress the interviewers than those who give obviously rehearsed and "coached" responses. There are clearly some questions which schools and students will anticipate (see below) but during the course of the interview there will be other questions which occur spontaneously to the interviewers and cannot be anticipated by the students.

Why do you want to be a doctor
This is an obvious though vital question. It is also the question to which candidates most frequently reply with a coached and

practised answer. Rehearsed answers do not rule a candidate out of consideration, however they are clearly not as impressive as answers which are spontaneous and show genuine flair and enthusiasm for the subject.

Previous caring experience
Experience of a caring role will clearly be a topic raised by the interviewers. This role need not be in a traditional mainstream medical environment. The interview is an opportunity for candidates to relate not only the facts and details of their role but also their emotional response to it, what it has taught them, and what they have gained from it.

Matters of medical interest
Candidates will not be expected to have knowledge of details of medical processes. However, the panel will feel it reasonable to expect the candidate to have an intelligent lay person's view on many aspects of medicine particularly those of current media interest.

Ethical issues
Ethical issues may be raised by the interview panel but only in so far as to assess the candidate's ability to coherently summarise the issues at stake. Candidates should be reassured that neither the panel nor the Medical School will take a position on any ethical issue. It is not the candidate's ethical views that the panel may be interested in but how coherently the candidate expresses the ethical dilemmas facing medical practitioners. Candidates will not be asked questions in any of the following areas: gender, sexuality, marital or parental status, race, religion, social background.

Decisions

At the end of the interview, after each candidate has left the room, the panel will discuss his/her merits for approximately five minutes. Candidates will not be informed of the decision of the panel on the day of the interview. Candidates will receive the University's decision by post. All offers are conditional upon the achievement of the appropriate standard in forthcoming examinations (if the candidate has not already satisfied our academic requirements for entry) and upon completion of health screening and clearance by the Criminal Record Bureau.

Interview 1
Why Manchester?
What part of course attracted you?
What else about PBL?
Why Medicine?
What would you do if part of the team wasn't pulling their weight?
Who is responsible for sorting this out?
What do you do to relax?
Do you think it is stressful for a doctor
Why?
How would you cope?
Will it be easy for you to cope?
Questions related to work experience
What do you think will be the advancements in medicine in the next 20 years?
What are the bad points about being a doctor
How would you protect yourself from litigation?
What factors affected the health of Victorians?
What differences do you think there will be when you're a doctor
Who would you put on a panel to discuss Gene Therapy?
How do you relax?

Interview 2
Why medicine?
How would you deal with mistakes?
What do you know about the course?
What do you think of PBL?
What would you do if someone wasn't pulling their weight?
What are the major developments in medicine in the last 20 years?
What about the MMR vaccine?

Should Tony Blair disclose statistics regarding surgeons success rates?
What developments do you expect in the next 20 years?
What about cloning?
What do you think would improve the NHS if you were in charge what would you do to improve it?

Interview 3
Why Manchester?
What are disadvantages of PBL?
Why Medicine?
What stresses are doctors under?
How do you cope with stress?
What do you see as being the advancements of the near future?
What would you say you have learnt about medicine from working in a hospice?

Interview 4
My medicine and not nursing?
Why Manchester?
Tell us a bit about PBL.....any advantages?
How would you encourage your PBL group to work?
What if someone really wasn't contributing at all?
What other reasons for choosing Manchester
What would you do if you made a mistake, resulting in the death of a patient
How would you get over the death/ deal with it?
Loads about communication!!
A bit about genetics (related to my P.S.)
A bit about S. America (P.S. related again)
How would you get the balance between work/leisure?
How would I cope with the long hours?
Briefly How was your journey? train/car?
So why do you want to study Medicine , why not other related careers?

Interview 5

There are Medical schools near you, so why have you applied to Manchester?
What do you know about PBL ?, It has been criticised recently so what are the disadvantages of it?
Why would a person not be committed to his set PBL group?
How do you cope with stress?
How do you think you will cope with stress being a doctor
So you have done lots of experience, Do you remember any particular patient that you met or saw? (My answer was about an old lady that didn't reply to me when I asked her what she wanted for lunch)
Why do you think she didn't answer you?
Did you ask the nurse what was wrong with her?
Case : Should a man with lung cancer from smoking be treated or a man with lung cancer not caused by smoking?
What if the finance was limited?
Who to spend the money to treat?
Who decides who will receive the treatment?

Interview 6
Why do you want be a doctor
Why not a nurse or physiotherapist or dentist?
How do you cope with stress?
What would you do if a mother didn't want her child to get the MMR? What is herd immunity?
Extra curricular activities?
Student life and work?

Interview 7
1) Why did you decide to do medicine?
2) What made you choose Manchester medical school?
3) Why medicine and not nursing or dentistry?
4) If you were part of a team and one person wasn't doing any work and the another was too expressive in their opinions, how would you deal with this?
5) Do you think medicine is a science or an art??

6) What would you do as team building exercises?
(I talked about more socialising and involving everyone...
Slipped in a comment about the sports facilities at the university)
7) How would you deal with a great workload/?

Interview 8
1) From your personal statement you say you did some work experience
in a hospital in a 3rd world country. What were the similarities and differences compared to Britain?
2) What do you think is the hardest job for a doctor in a hospital and a G.P.?
3) If you had the worst day, you re patient died and you come home at
3:00 am..what would you do to unwind and de-stress?
4) how would you manage with all the stress and how would you
Keep yourself motivated for so long?

Interview 9
1) How far do you think medical soaps on TV educate the public on Preventative medicine?
2) Do you think more should be done to make these dramas realistic?
3) Recently there was a story line where a man needed an organ transplant and the only way to get this was to kill a live man. What do you think of this?
4) Killing people for donors happens often in 3rd world countries? Why do you think this?
5) What topic would you like to see more of in medical soaps?

Interview 10

 Should NHS pay for plastic surgery?
You are a G.P. of a child that is very unhappy because she is bullied about her ears. Would you refer her for a plastic surgery?
What did you enjoy most about your work experience?

What do you do in your free time to relax?
What did you like best about Duke of Edinburgh Award?
Could you describe a situation in which you acted as a leader?
Do you prefer to be a leader or follow others?
What are the disadvantages of being a doctor

Interview 11
Why medicine
Why Manchester
What are limitations of pbl
Do I think pbl would have helped interviewer when she was studying medicine
Would I carry on with my extra curricular activities if I came to Manchester and why is it important to me
Differences between NHS and private
Duke of Edinburgh... what did I find out about myself... any lows... put it in medical context
General conversation on advertising on a whole
Drugs.. Good and bad points
McDonalds KFC and stuff
Control of advertising on media internet

Interview 12
How was your journey, did you travel far etc
What did you like about man to make you apply here?
What attracted to you about man (talked about PBL, loved the city, personal stuff etc)
Advantages of pbl
We are doctors and we learned medicine the "old school" method via lectures, do you think that puts us at a disadvantage?
Why medicine
What were the highlights for you from your work experience that made you decide to do medicine
Negative aspects of medicine
Then for 5 mins at the end we talked about should alcohol be banned to reduce binge drinkers.

Interview 13
How was your journey?
Why medicine?
The things you've described could be applied to a career in psychology too why not psychology?
Why Manchester?
What attributes do you have that would make you suited to a PBL course?
If you found that one person in your PBL group was not pulling their weight, what do you think you should do?
You said on your PS that you worked on a project in Romania could you tell us about it?
What did you take away from the experience?
Tell us about your work experience?
What is your opinion on plastic surgery being offered on the NHS?
How should it be decided who should qualify for such surgery?
Who should decide generally how the NHS spends money?
Why not the general public?

Interview 14

What aspects of your job as an optometrist will make you a better doctor
Why move away from optometry?
How will you cope with the work load?
What do you to relax?
Give an example when you've had to overcome something difficult.
Bits about work experience, what have you done, examples of specific scenarios etc.
Then a 'discussion', which is paraphrased from 'a series of ridiculous questions' about plastic surgery on the NHS. This was tough but hopefully I came across okay.

Only 15 minutes, goes fast.

Interview 15
When did you decided you wanted to be a doctor
What specific experiences has lead you here?
What are the ups and downs of being a doctor
How will you cope with the course?
How will you cope with the stress of the job?
What do you do to relax?

Then the ethical discussion:
Should plastic surgery be available on the NHS?
Who makes the decisions and how and why?

Interview 16

Why medicine and not dentistry?
How do you cope with stress?
What would you do if a consultant shouted at you for making a mistake?
What do you to do relax?
Tell us about the course?
What possible problems might you face as a doctor in 20 years time?
What changes in the last 50 years or so have affected the health of the nation?
If I could put together a ethical committee about genetic engineering, who would I put on it?
What recent medical article had I read?
What was the most significant medical breakthrough in the last century?
Tell us about PBL?
You say the students like it, why do they like it?
If someone in a PBL group wasn't pulling their weight what would you do?
How do you cope with stress?
What have been the major public health advances of the last 50 yrs.?
What have you read in the medical press in the last 5 yrs. that has interested you?

What do you think about stem cell research?
Bits about my hobbies in between to try and relax me.... Didn't work!

Newcastle, University of, The Medical School

Interview 1
It was very short lasted only 10 mins so you really have to think on your feet!
I got asked about religious views in medicine and whether or not I thought they were important.
About problems with the NHS and that if I had control of the funds what would I do with them.
Then general things about myself, extra curricular etc and about things I said in my personal statement, so be prepared to explain things you have written.

Interview 2
Why doctor
Why Newcastle? (In terms of the course structure)
Do you think you're a good listener?
What qualities do you have that'll make you a good doctor
If you were the senior health officer in with a pot of gold, what would you do with it?
What has been your biggest challenge in life?
What do you do in spare time?
What can you bring to the university? (sports etc)

Nottingham, The University of, Faculty of Medicine and Health Sciences

Interview 1
Two interviewers, 20 minutes, Interview after Christmas informed within 12 weeks.
How did you get to Nottingham? Who did you come with. Have you done anything interesting in the last few days.

Why did you choose Nottingham and why also Neuroscience (back up choice)?
Have you read anything medically related recently? This lead to further discussion. Have you read anything medically related in the national press recently.

Ethical issue; whether to be honest with the public and sacrifice a friendship with a colleague by admitting her mistake or conceal it.

Interview 2

15 min interview with a male and female interviewer. Tour at 11.00, interviews 1.30-4.30. I went in 45 min. because they were ahead of schedule so it is worth being in the waiting area early

How did you get here today?
Why Nottingham?
And?
And?!
Why medicine?
What have you seen of doctors at work?
What did you gain from your work experience?
Give me an example of a time when you have shown empathy.
How do you cope with stress
What skills do you think you need to be a good doctor
Any questions?

Interview 3
Why do you want to be a doctor
What are qualities that good doctors should have?
Which of these do you have?
Are there any of these qualities or other factors that you feel you will need to improve to become a good doctor
Why Nottingham?
What interests you about this course over the newer PBL courses?
How do you feel about getting the BMedSci after 3 years?

How will the skills learn during this help you in your role as a doctor

Interview 4
Why medicine?
Why Nottingham?
What makes Nottingham different from other medical schools?
Why did I take Geography A-Level?
What medical news has caught your attention recently? Then questions on stem cells
Why Nottingham should choose me over other candidates?
What difficulties does a doctor face?

Interview 5
Why medicine?
How will your pharmacy studies help you?
Pros and cons of cannabis decriminalisation?
Why do youngsters use cannabis?
How will you cope with students younger than you?
How do you make patients feel comfortable?
What do you do to relax?
What are the bad points of being a doctor
Work/experience
What do you think about the effects of the media's negative reporting on the profession?
Why Nottingham?

Interview 6
"Why do you want to be a Doctor"
"What personal qualities do you have?"
"What makes a good doctor"
"Give me some health disciplines."
"What particularly appeals to you about the course at Nottingham?"
"There are a lot of good candidates, why should we offer you the place?"
"Tell us about an interesting scientific article that you've read recently."

"What are your hobbies?"
"What did you learn from your work experience?"
"What would you do if you were the health secretary?"
"What problems do doctors face in the future?"
"What are your weaknesses?"

Interview 7
How are your other applications going?
Is Nottingham your first choice?
What do you think is the purpose of including a second degree in a medical course?
Why medicine?
What qualities should a doctor have?
What are the good things about being a doctor
Are there any bad things?
Have you encountered any terminally ill or difficult patients?
Do you read about current medical issues?
What recent medical topic can you tell us about?
What do you do to relax?
How did you hear about the course and university
What would you expect to be learning considering it is a systems based course.
What do you like about the course
How did your parents influence you (both are doctors)
Talk to us about something medical that interests you.
What would you do in the 3rd year of the course...(BMedSci)
What happens in the third year?

Suggest the benefits of doing a research project
Questions on work experience seemed to go on forever!
Questions on hobbies
Pressures of being a doctor
How do you relax?
Supposing you were Milburn's right hand man, which policies would you suggest should be introduced?
How can we improve the current state of the NHS?

What is welfare like for the elderly? Which problems arise? Why do these problems arise?
How would you break bad news to a patient?

Interview 8
What is good about the course?
Why is having a BSc an advantage?
What do you like about the method of learning?
Why should we pick you? What would you do for the university?
What are the advantages and disadvantages of being a doctor
What do you think about euthanasia?
Are there any good reasons for euthanasia today?
Do you get to read much out of school about medical topics?
Do you know what oncology is?
What's asperger's syndrome?
Did you try to get hospital work experience?
What did you see during your work shadowing?

Interview 9
What do you think makes a good doctor and why would you make a good doctor
Apparently I kept mentioning the doctor and 'HIS team' so they asked can you think of when the doctor isn't the most important person in the team?
They kept pushing that question and I wasn't entirely sure what they were getting at!
Why Nottingham?
What do you do to keep up to date with medical advances?
What was the last thing you read in the newspaper/medical journal?
What do you think we should allow medical students to do so that they get a proper insight into the medical career..
I've run out of questions now, have you got any for me?

Interview 10

Why medicine?

What are the qualities of a good doctor
What are the bad aspects of being a doctor
Why Nottingham?
What makes a good friend?
Give an example to show you are a good friend?
Qualities you possess which makes you think you would make a good doctor
Your friend's parents have just got divorced. He comes to you for help. How do you react/what do you do?

Interview 11
Why Nottingham?
What is the advantage of a Doctor in having a background in research?
What is more important research or treating patients?
Lots of questions on work experience.
From your work experience what do think you prefer to go into; general practice, hospital medicine or surgery?
Why is a G.P.s role important?
Why does a G.P. need to have good communication skills?
Why did you chose to do the OU human genome course?
What is the role of a Doctor
Dissection its a bit barbaric isn't it?!
Negative aspects of medicine?
How do you cope with stress?

Interview 12

Why medicine?
Why Nottingham?
Work experience?
Why do you think having the extra BSc is an advantage?
But when I see an application I only look to see that they have a medical degree. Why else do you think its helpful/useful?
How do you think surgeons are assessed?
Do you really think that is the best way?

Then I got asked about alzheimers, and why people say if they could find a drug to delay the onset by 5 years then it would be a lot better and a cure wouldn't need to be found.

Attributes Oxford University look for at interview

Personal characteristics: suitability for medicine
- Empathy: ability and willingness to imagine the feelings of others and understand the reasons for the views of others
- Motivation: a reasonably well informed and strong desire to practise medicine
- Communication: ability to make knowledge and ideas clear using language appropriate to the audience
- Honesty and Integrity
- Ethical awareness
- Ability to work with others
- Capacity for sustained and intense work

Academic Potential
- Problem solving: critical thinking, analytical approach
- Intellectual curiosity: keenness to understand the reason for observations; depth; tendency to look for meaning; enthusiasm and curiosity in science
- Communication skills: willingness and ability to express clearly and effectively; ability to listen; compatibility with tutorial format

Peninsula Medical school

You will receive an introductory talk about the selection process. You are then asked to complete a questionnaire that explores your commitment and motivation to do medicine. You are then given three ethical scenarios related to medicine, one of which you select as the basis for your interview. The interview is 20 minutes and all candidates are asked the same questions and given the same prompts. They are looking for communication and listening skills. Potential for both leadership and team player. Ability to deal with stress, problem solving skills, veracity and honesty empathy ability to be non judgmental reflective and awareness of your limitations.

Interview 1
15 minute interview with 3 interviewers doctor, admissions officer, nurse. Interview Questions were based on an ethical scenario for which I was given 20 minutes preparation time. Questions included:
"If you were a doctor in this situation, what would you do?"
"What are the ethical implications in this situation? For who? You as a doctor The patient?"
"How do doctors cope with stress?"
"Give an example of when you worked in a team?"
"Give an example of a difficult situation you encountered? How did you solve the problem?"
20 minute questionnaire given prior to interview. Questions included:
"What attributes do you have to make you a good doctor"
"Why do you want to come to this medical school?"
"What problems are currently impacting on the NHS?"
30 minute group exercise with 6 other candidates. We were given a non medical topic to discuss, and had to weigh up the advantages and the disadvantages of the situation.
Tips
Find out about the moral and ethical duties of a doctor
Be prepared to answer questions about yourself honestly
Be friendly and relaxed
Other comments
Interviewers were friendly and did not grill me about medical topics. Before the interview, we were given the opportunity to talk to current medical students, so feel free to ask them questions
Research the medical school beforehand, as interviewers want to know why you want to come to this particular institution.

The University of Sheffield, School of Medicine

Why medicine?

Why Sheffield?
Do you know Sheffield well?
Do you see it as an advantage that you live fairly close?
What qualities should a doctor have that you possess?
I talked about teamwork as one of my points and mentioned Duke of Edinburgh, so they said 'Tell us about D of E'.
What do you do to relax?
Tell us about a story in medicine you have read recently.
Any questions?
Then the consultant suddenly asked when I thought it was all over:
Do you have any beliefs that would affect the way you practice?

University of Southampton, School of Medicine

Do not interview

University of Swansea, Swansea Clinical School

Questions were asked which focused on the personal statement.
Then 'why do you want to be a doctor/what makes a good doctor',

Ethical scenario where I, as a doctor, have killed someone who otherwise would have survived how would I deal with that/what do I tell family
What have you accomplished ?
What do you regard as your major non academic achievement
Why do you need a challenging career
You want to help people so why not become a nurse
What are your limitations
Describe yourself (6 good and 6 bad)
Why should we give you a place

University College Medical School of University College London

Interview 1

Why medicine?
What pressures are put on doctors?
As a doctor, how would you overcome these pressures? What pressures are there on medicine as a whole?
Tell us about one patient you met during your work experience that stood out to you.
How could that patients care have been made better?
Imagine you are a doctor You have a male patient who is married and has a family. You have just had results back that confirm he is HIV+, what are you going to do?
Your next patient dies because you made a mistake, what are you going to do?
Why aren't you taking biology A level?
Is psychology an art or a science?
Tell me about the differences between medical practice in America (where I did some work experience) and here.
Why did you apply to Cardiff?
How will you cope with the stresses of medicine?
What have you heard from your other three choices?
What would you spend £50 on if I were to give it to you for tonight?
What are your views on the Phillips paper
You're the first person I've met to have worked in a hospice what did you learn there?

Interview 2
What have you heard form everywhere else you've applied to?
How do you relax?
How do you deal with stressful situations/'difficult' customers?
What would you do if something went wrong?
Tell us about a recent medical advance you have read about in the newspapers.
What area are you most interested in?
What out of school interests do you have?
Details of work experience.

What makes a good doctor what qualities?

Interview 3
I understand you have had work experience at a general practice and at a hospital, what were the differences between the two placements?
What are the qualities of a good doctor
Why do you want to study medicine?
I have heard that you read science journals. Is there anything that you have read that has struck you?
Do you believe what you read was a break through?
I read here that your father is a doctor You have obviously had an insight of a career of medicine from one side? Did this influence you to take a career in medicine?
What did you learn from your work experience?
Did everyone go home after being treated at the ward you were working at?
What do you do to relax?
In what area do you think you'd like to specialise?
What percentage of a doctor's work is just social work?
If you were health secretary what would you do to improve the NHS?
Would a huge pay rise for medical staff help?
What would you do about improving the organisation of the NHS?

Interview 4
What have you gained from working with disabled people?
If a child was in need of surgery and the parents were being extremely demanding, what would you do?
Tell us about your work experience and what did you learn from it? Do you think it was beneficial
What do you know about variant CJD? It will soon be standard practice to screen blood donors for vCJD. If you found that a potential donor was vCJD positive would you tell them and why?
How does the government find out about problems and issues in the NHS?
I see you are a beach lifeguard. Does this involve regular training and

updating of your skills?
I see here, you worked at an old people's home, what did you learn about people??
What pressures are there on doctors?
They asked something which drew on from my answer about doctors not getting too emotionally involved.....and asked "what do you mean doctors shouldn't get emotionally involved with patients?"
I see here you were chosen to be school captain....tell me why you think you were elected?
I see here you are doing an AS in ICT? How do you think IT can help within medicine?
Asked me about evidence based learning and how is this helpful.

Interview 5
Have you always wanted to be a doctor When did you decide?
Why do you need a challenging career??
Tell me about a patient you saw on your work experience?
Why did this person stand out in your mind?
How did she get kidney failure?
Was she on insulin??
What type of art do you like?
What artist and why?
What do you think of Damien Hursts work and Tracey Emins?
Would you pay £500 for it?
How can art be used with disabled children?
What have you learnt most from your work experience?
How would you befriend a elderly person differently to a young one in hospital?
What do you think about doctor's private hours being restricted?
Why can't dialysis patient's dialyse at night?

Interview 6
How are you.
What articles have you read that are medically related. Mentioned cervical cancer vaccine and cloning.
What newspapers do you read, do you believe what the news papers

say.
Do you think cloning is a good idea.
I see that on your form you say you are dyslexic, how will this affect you as a medic.
Why now (as you are "quite" old)?
What I learned from my voluntary work.
Did I have a chance to spend much time with doctors while doing this?
What qualities do you think you can bring to medicine? Talked about communication skills and used an example of being an employee representative for a strategic review at work.
What I had learned from this about "management".
Questions about personal statement. My jobs since returning to UK 3 years ago. What I do in my current job.
How I think working for NHS would be different from working for a private sector company. Didn't really get the question they were talking about the frustrations of such a move.

Interview 7
What did you learn from your work experience?
What kind of patients were on the ward?
What did you learn from your voluntary work?
Were you always on the same ward?
Did you see the same patients more than once?
What did you gain from changing schools at sixth form?
How did you benefit from doing extracurricular activities at new school?
I see you visited body worlds, do you think it was right to display organs in that way
Question about CEP project we did in school..
Why diabetes ? We did the cep project on a health education booklet, on diabetes)
Did you do it on diabetes because incidence of diabetes in an Asian population is so high?
What percentage of people have diabetes?
What have you just studied in chemistry?

Interview 8
Why did you choose to take the International Baccalaureate?
Where do you see yourself in twenty years time?
What are the demands of a medical career?
Why should we take you?
Question related to kinetic theory... how temp affects rate..
Question on what we're learning in biology.
Question relating to biology work
Question about euthanasia, do you think its right?.
Question about organ trade, is it right for money?
What position do you play in rugby?
I see you speak French? Oui un peu, he didn't understand!
Is it a family thing?
Do you think people should sell organs?
Can you name any major markets in medicine?
Do you read news articles?
Tell me about the human genome project?
Do you think it is a good thing for people to know they will develop an illness.
You think it would give them peace of mind?
Name me prevalent conditions that have a genetic basis? Dementia, Cerebral Palsy (I forgot to say congenital heart disease, diabetes, cancer)
Do you have any question for us?

Interview 9

Questions about voluntary work and what I do
You seem very busy, yet you play football every day...
What do you think you can bring to UCL?
Did you think the BMAT essay was a good idea? What's Amnesty's stance on organ donation?
One thing that shocked you during your work experience
Did this not put you off medicine?
What do you think is the biggest problem facing medicine in the

21st century?

Interview 10
What do you think you can bring to UCL?
Did you think the BMAT essay was a good idea?
What's Amnesty's stance on organ donation?
If all available organs weren't working what would you do?
I think you misunderstood, have you heard of organ rejection and how this occurs?
You mentioned the heart attack patient you saw earlier. How does this happen?
What can be done to treat this?
If this was unavailable what could you do alternatively?)
Any questions?

Interview 11
What qualities make a good doctor, and which of these qualities do you think you possess?
At your work experience did you see all these skills, give us an example. Who else did you talk to at you work experience?
What recent medical advancements have you read about?
What have you read that tells you about medicine as a career?
Consider this example; The government is considering giving all doctors guidelines for all cases. Should this protocol always be followed in all cases? Should doctors ever have to think outside the box?
How would you deal with not being able to complete a form of treatment because of inadequate funding?
Why did you go to radiology in your work experience? Were you considering that as a possible career path?
They asked me to speak about Theology A level what it involves why I did it and how it is relevant to medicine
Spoke about new drinking laws + whether it was good or bad, and to approach it also from an ethical point of view
Spoke about smoking regulations how was it fair we use to be able to only drink until say 11, but could smoke whenever, even though

passive smoking effects the people around you but drinking doesn't.
Asked me how I dealt with pressure
Asked me a little bit about my work experience

Interview 12
So I see you've volunteered in a nursery, why do you want to become a doctor and not a nursery teacher?
How do you relax? What do you do to relax?
What would you do on a long plane journey?
What would you read if I locked you up in a house for a week?
Why UCL?
Questions about the BMAT essay I wrote.
What advantage does playing the viola have over playing the violin?
Why did you choose to apply for medicine instead of music?
BMAT questions: Can you summarise the main arguments in your essay?
Is that really what you mean?
Interviewer asked me whether I think clean drinking water for all is more important than medicine for all the sick then decided that it was a difficult question to answer
If you had limited resources in a hospital, how would you choose which SARS patients to admit?
How do you plan to pay for your medical education?

Interview 13
Why do you want to be a doctor
Why not a nurse?
What qualities do you think a doctor should have?
Do you have these qualities?
Tell me about (insert hobby)
What sort of illnesses did you see at your work experience?
Follow on questions about MRSA (what I saw, what is it etc)
Tell me about differences in health care in England and Bahrain (where I did some work experience)
You shadowed X what did you see that was interesting, was there a patient that stood out to you?

You wake up tomorrow and you are the minister of health, what changes would you make to the NHS?
Should there be a limit on how much funding the NHS should receive?
What is that limit?
More questions about hobbies.
Then, your BMAT essay discussed patient confidentiality with minors.
When would there be a cause to break confidentiality of an adult? Who would you break it to?
When would you involve the family (because I said the reason could be threatening to commit suicide)
When would you involve the police..would you at all?
Do you think people with self inflicted diseases such as obesity, alcoholism should be refused treatment?
You play piano, how's that going?

Interview 14
Why do you want to do medicine?
How is it that you developed your interest in the body?
Tell me about a recent problem about funding in the NHS (talked about herceptin but in hindsight I think he may well have been asking about pfi)
Tell me about what you saw on work experience
You also spent some time with your G.P., did you talk to any of the patients there?
Give me an example of where a doctor would have to tell a partner about his patient
Who can doctors go to discuss such problems?
So you volunteer with children, what exactly do you do there? How did this boy with learning difficulties become like that?

Interview 15
In your statement you say you have developed the skill of report writing and that this is important in being a doctor, why?
If you had to reduce the NHS drug budget, where would you start?

You said you've seen a bone marrow biopsy, describe it.
What was the last non academic book you read? What was it about?
What do you think will be the most difficult thing to deal with as a doctor How will you cope with it?
How will you cope with stress?
Where do you see yourself in 15 years?
Asked about the entry exam essay FMAT you talk about 'well established theories' , why did you use the word theory rather than idea?
Your father is a doctor, is that why you want to study medicine?
Talk about some recent medical news.
What is your favourite subject and why?

Interview 16

These are the comments as reported by one prospective student verbatim.

I had an interview at UCL on the 15th December, a day before my 18th birthday. It was horrific, I've always been quite a confident speaker but they argued every point that I made and made me stick up for every answer I gave. They also wouldn't let me answer questions about myself with – 'I think I am…'. However 3 days later I received an offer of AAB thus am very happy.
The interview was 15 minutes long and the panel consisted of 2 doctors and a student, only the doctors spoke.
What are your selfish reasons for wanting to be a Doctor?
Do you regret the 1st line of your personal statement? (My wish to study medicine was confirmed the first time I gave blood it thrilled and humbled me that my blood could help, or even save, someone.)
Do you think that blood donation and organ donation should be compulsory?
10 years only 2% of graduate medical students thought that medicine was the same as any other job, now 8% think so' what do you think and why has there been this change?
How would you encourage a 13 year old to take RS GCSE or would

you alternatively try to dissuade her?
Sell yourself to us in 1minute (I am sure that it was more than one minute)
You now have 5 minutes to ask us questions…

Interview 17
Are you sure that a course in Medicine would be satisfying for you to undergo as your Academic profile would suggest that a straight single discipline course would be more suitable for you?
Would you have problems identifying with people from a different socioeconomic background to yourself?"
"What is your opinion on "Widening access to Medicine courses?"
Why medicine?
What qualities in a good doctor
Give an example when you worked as a team leader/player
Have you ever had to make an important/difficult decision as a team leader?
Who is the most important person in a medical team?
Is research important? Then talk about recent research you have read about

St George's University of London

Qualities of a Doctor
What did you learn from your work experience?
Advantages and disadvantages of working in medicine? Didn't talk about ethical issues.
A recent article you have read about/research in medicine?
A difficult situation/ an example of a difficult issue in your life and how you dealt with it?
What do you do to relax? And why do you think it is important to relax when working in medicine?
And after some of these questions, anything else, anything else.

George's are basing a lot of emphasis on ones Personal statements this year, so the best piece of advice would be to know it very well!!

In addition they tend to have typical questions such as:

What qualities do doctor's need to have and do you possess any of them?
How do you make decisions?…Which may be further followed by; give an example of when you have had to make the most difficult decision?
Recent research paper that you have read and why it interested you?
For graduates they often tend to ask why research is important and what are the negative aspects of research?
Why George's and what would you offer George's if we give you a place?
Is a Doctor a leader or a follower? Which one are you???
How do you deal with conflict?

What do you think you could contribute to this medical school
Sell yourself to us in 2 minutes

A collection of additional questions previously used in interviews

Motivation for medicine

Why do you believe you have the ability to undertake the study and work involved?
Why do you want to study medicine?
What do you think being a doctor entails?
What branch of medicine do you think would interest you? Why?
How do you think medicine differs from other health professions?
Do you have any work experience that has given you insight into the work of medicine?
When you think about becoming a doctor, what do you look forward to most and least?

What impact do you hope to make in the field of medicine?
What one question would you ask if interviewing others interested in studying medicine?
Why study medicine rather than any other health care profession?
What aspect of health care attracts you to medicine?
Why do you want to be a doctor
What steps have you taken to try to find out whether you really do want to become a doctor
This course will require a good deal of independent study, how have you managed this approach to learning in the past?
What things do you think might make people inclined to drop out of medical training?
There are many different ways of helping people. Why do you

What have you read or experienced that you feel has particularly prepared you for medicine?
Why do you want to be a doctor
Why not a nurse?
What have you accomplished
What do you regard as your major non academic achievement
Why do you need a challenging career
Have you always wanted to be a doctor
You want to help people so why not become a nurse
What are your limitations
Describe yourself (6 good and 6 bad)
Why should we give you a place
What do you think you could contribute to this medical school
Sell yourself to us in 2 minutes
Why medicine
Why are you suited to medicine
· What qualities would you regard as essential for a doctor
What qualities in a doctor are missing in you & do you think you can improve them
What have you read or experienced that you feel has particularly prepared you for medicine?
Why do you want to study medicine, rather than working in any

other health or social care professions?
There are many ways of helping people. Why do you want to do this through medicine?
What do you hope to achieve as a doctor
What would you most like us to ask you in this interview?
Tell me what you have learnt from a medical or scientific project (or from work experience) you have undertaken?

Depth and breadth of interest
Can you tell me about a significant recent advance in medicine or science?
What do you consider to be the most important advances in medicine over the last 50/ 100 years?
What do you think is the future outlook of our planet?
What medical stories are significant in the media at the moment?
Tell us about some issues in the history of medicine that interest you.
How do you think you will avoid problems of keeping up to date during a long career?
What movie have you seen, recently, that has made you think and why?
What do you think is the most important medical discovery in the last 100 200 years, and why?
Tell me about a book or a film that has influenced you and why?

Tell me about someone who has been a major influence on your life?
What do you think was the greatest public health advance of the twentieth century?
What do you think about David Blaine?
Will you please describe an interesting place you have been to, and explain why it was so?
Will you please tell me about an interesting experience, and what you learned from it?
How important is it to be up to date? How will you cope with not always being up to date?
Tell me about some medical press stories you have read recently.
Tell me about a non academic project or piece of organisation that

you were involved in. How did it go?
What would (will) you do in a gap year? Why?
Tell me about a medical problem or technique you have seen in the media recently?

Team work
What groups would you imagine working with in your role as a doctor
Who do you think is the most important member of a multi disciplinary health care team? Why?
What are the advantages and disadvantages of being in a team?
How do you think you would cope with criticism from colleagues or other health professionals?
Modern day health care is very much a team effort. Could you give an example of a role that you have played in a team and
what you contributed?
What do you think of nurses developing extended roles and undertaking tasks previously done by doctors?
What do you think about the proposal that nurses could replace doctors as the first contact person in primary care?
When you are a doctor you will be working in a team. Who will you include in your team, and why?
What makes a good team member & what have you noticed about working in a team
Have you ever been a leader, what does it involve
Give examples where you have used teamwork and leadership skills
Do you prefer being a team leader or a team worker
· Comment on teamwork and communication skills
What do you understand by the term good health
How important is teamwork?

Personal Insight
What experience do you have of people with medical conditions/ in health care environments?
Have you visited any friends or family in hospital? What did you see that you would like to change?

What are your outside interests and hobbies?

Tell us two personal qualities you have which would make you a good doctor

Tell us about two personal shortcomings that you think you would like to overcome as you become doctor

Some doctors who qualify never practice. What makes you think you will stick to it?

What do you think will be the most difficult things you might encounter during your study?

What relevance to medicine are the 'A' levels (apart from biology and chemistry) that you have been studying?

What skills do you think are needed in order to communicate with your patients; how do you think they are best acquired?

If you were to become a doctor, how would you wish your patients to describe you and why?

What interests do you bring from school/college life that you think will contribute to your studies and practice?

Have there been any particular life experiences that you think will help you in a career in medicine?

What challenges do you think a career in medicine will bring you?

What do you think you will be the most positive aspects of being a doctor

What do you think you will be the most negative aspects of being a doctor How will you motivate yourself for the tedious parts?

What do you see as the disadvantages of being a doctor

What attributes are necessary in a good doctor

Thinking about yourself: what characteristics do you think you would most need to change in the course of becoming a good doctor

Medicine will bring you into contact with a vast range of different people, with different cultures, what experience have you had of different types of people?

If you could only tell me one thing about yourself, to help me to get a sense of you as a person, what would it be and why?

If you could change 1 or 2 things about yourself, what would it/they be?

Tell me about a difficult situation you have dealt with and what you

learned from it?
What do you think are your priorities in your own personal development?
What qualities do you lack that would be useful for a doctor, and what do you intend to do about this?
What qualities do you think other people value in you?
How do you think other people would describe you?

Coping with Stress

How do you cope with stress
What will you do if a person turns aggressive towards you
What would you do if a consultant shouted at you if you made a mistake
If you were attacked by a person while performing surgery what would you do
What possible problems might you face as a consultant in 20 years
How can being a G.P. be frustrating
What about the criticism of doctors nowadays
· What do you consider the main problems that confront doctors in training
You've encountered doctors during work experience; did they say anything about the bad aspects of medicine?
What have you noticed about working in a team?
What do you do to relax
How would you approach the uncertainties in medicine?
What's the down side of being a doctor And how would you cope with it?
What qualities do you look for in a doctor
How would you cope with the stress of being a doctor
 Can you think of an example where doctors were faced with a difficult decision? How would you go about it?
What possible problems might you face as a doctor in 20 years time
 Give example of having to use communication skills in a tough situation
Do you read, what kind of books/newspapers

Who is your favourite artist
? What good qualities do you have that you can bring to medicine
You say you can speak other languages, how would that be useful in studying or practising medicine?
Do you think you'll be able to carry on with your hobbies at university?
What do you do in your spare time?
Do you think it's important for a doctor to have outside interests
What do you do to relax?
How do you cope in situations where there is not enough time to finish a task?
We all know exams are stressful. How did you manage when you were taking your GCSEs?
What do you do when you have 3 or 4 things to do that are all urgent?
Evidence of working both as a leader and team member; ability to multi task:
Have you dealt with a difficult situation?
I see you are captain of a team. What duties does that involve?
How do you feel about sharing work with others?
How do you balance work and all your outside activities?
I see you play sport/do the Duke of Ed/play in the orchestra (or similar) why is this important to you?
I see you were Director/Manager in your Young Enterprise company. How did you go about performing this role

Knowledge of Medical training and why this course?

What do you know about self directed learning
What area would you like to specialise in and why?
· Tell us about the course
What diseases would you like to study with our resources
Limitations of PBL/self directed learning
Who do you register with after PRHO year
What do GMC and RCS mean
·· Where do you see yourself in 10 years

What do you want to specialise in
Are there exams after university, what are they
Describe the path after medical school
· Where do you see yourself in 10 years time?
Which medical professional do you admire the most?
What, in particular attracts you to study at X?
Tell us what attracts you most and least about the X Medical School
What ways of working and studying have you developed that you think will assist you through medical school?
Why have you chosen X rather than other medical schools?
What do you understand by PBL?
What are the advantages of a PBL course?
Why do you want to come to a PBL medical school?
Why do you think a PBL course will suit you personally?
What do you know about the course in Hull/York?
Why do you want to come to a new medical school?
What interests you about X School?
Why do you think problem based learning will suit you?
What do you understand by a PBL medical course?
What is it that interests you most about coming to a new medical school?
What interests you about the curriculum?
When you read the prospectus, what appealed to you or interested you in the course here?

Understanding of the role of medicine in society and ethical issues

What problems do the elderly encounter
How would you act around an elderly person you know if they found out they were terminally ill
What diseases should be resourced more
What changes in the last 50 years have affected the health or the nation
Talk about a medical/ethical issue that you've seen in the media that's caught your attention
(Euthanasia, designer babies, cloning, religious issues e.g. Jehovah's

witnesses & transfusion)
Bristol babies scandal was seen as a learning curve, what is your opinion
Have you heard about the human genome project
What recent medical breakthroughs have risen
Which medical documentaries have you seen recently
What do you know about MMR
Advances in medicine in the last 5/20/50/100 years
What was the most significant breakthrough in the last century
What do you think will be at the cutting edge of medicine in the next 20 years
Comment on the role of hospital management
Computer use in health care
· When was the NHS founded
How has the NHS revolutionised medicine
Who was the 1st NHS minister
Comment on the conflict between NHS and the government
·4 things to mark the 50th anniversary of the NHS
Any dramatic changes since it was founded
Should we be made to pay for health care
Do you know how different the health system is in e.g. France
Comment on health care in developing countries
What do you think the NHS will be like in the future
If I gave you 10 million pounds for the NHS what would you do
Suggest how to reduce the costs of the NHS
If you were Mr. Hutton what changes would you make to the NHS
What were the most recent NHS reforms
Consultants contract why did they turn down a 24% increase
What do you think about doctor's private practice being curtailed
If you were prime minister what 3 government policies would you set to achieve
If you were to put together an ethical committee about genetic engineering who would you put on it
Why is research important
· Do you think doctors make a difference to national health
·

What health problems are encountered in east London, general health of local population

What did you think of Body worlds & do you think Prof Van Hagen did an autopsy for money

Who is your medical hero/who do you admire in the field of medicine

Do you think funding should be given to beggars and the homeless/would you give money directly to beggars and why

What recent stories have been in the press about medicine?

What would you do if you were in the ICU and had an elderly patient and the nurse told you that you are doing more damage by keeping them alive?

What do you know about MMR?

Do you think patient's view doctors as arrogant?

Is the NHS a good thing?

Why do we need screening and how do we carry it out.

What was the most significant medical breakthrough in the last century?

What changes in the last 50 years or so have affected the health of the nation?

What diseases should be resourced more?

How can medicine be implemented into social awareness?

Should politics influence health care provision? Why?

Some people say that practising medicine is as art. What do you understand by this?

Would you argue that medicine is a science or an art, and why?

Why do you think we hear so much about doctors and the NHS in the media today?

In what ways do you think doctors can promote good health?

Do you think doctors get a bad press, and if so, why?

Why do you think people are ready to criticise doctors and the NHS?

From what you have read and found out, where do you see the health service going?

What would you like to change about the current structure of the NHS?

Should infertility treatment be available on the NHS?

What do you see as government priorities in health care? What does the current government think our nation needs to focus on in terms of health?

How should the health service achieve a balance between promoting good health, and in treating ill health?

What do you think are the similarities and differences between being a doctor today and being a doctor 100 years ago?

What do equal opportunities mean to you, and does it affect the way you interact with others?

Do you think doctors have a right to strike?

Do you think patient's treatments should be limited by the NHS budget or do they have the right to new therapies no matter what the cost?

What does the term 'inequalities in health' mean to you?

How do you think the patient population will vary between Hull and York?

Do you think medicine should be more about changing behaviour to prevent disease or treating existing disease?

What do you think is the purpose of the health service in the 21st century?

If you were to design a booklet telling 12 year olds about being a doctor, what would you include?

What do you think are the chief difficulties faced by doctors in their work?

Everyone knows that doctors treat ill people. What else do you think doctors do?

If a benefactor offered you a huge amount of money to set up a Medical Research Institute and invited you to become its director, what research area would you choose to look at, and why?

Why do you think people in the north of England live, on average, 5 years less than those in the south?

What are the arguments for and against people paying for their own health care as and when they need it?

Do you think patients should pay to see the doctor

What do you understand by the term 'holistic' medicine?

How accurately do you think the media (particularly television) tend to portray the role of the doctor

Where does the most significant medical treatment take place?

What do you think is the greatest threat to the health of the British population today?

Have antibiotics or public health measures led to the most improvements in the nation's health?

Imagine you are on committee that has to recommend which of two new treatments can be made available through the NHS. On what grounds would you make your arguments?

Which is more important general practice (primary care) or hospital, and why?

Do you think euthanasia should be legalised? Discuss the pros and cons.

Do you think the country needs more doctors or more nurses?

What are the arguments for and against banning the sale of tobacco?

What do you think will be the effects of having more female doctors than male doctors?

Should life be prolonged at all costs?

Why do doctors sometimes get a bad press?

In some cases, NHS fertility treatment / cosmetic surgery is refused because patients smoke / are obese what do you think about this and why?

What is meant by the inequalities of health and what can be done to reduce them?

You have two patients, a 70 year old man who has had a heart attack and a 17 year old man who has had a motorbike accident, both of whom need intensive care beds. However, you only have one bed. Who do you give it to?

Can you tell us of any recent medical stories you've seen or read about?

Evidence of commitment to caring/ tolerance of ambiguity Work Experience

What aspect of your work experience did you find the most and least

interesting, and why?
In your work experience, what skills have you learnt that you can apply to medicine?
Can you give me an example of how you coped with a difficult situation with a colleague or friend; what strategy did you use and why?
Reflect on what you have seen of hospitals or a health care environment. What would you most like to organise differently, and why?
What aspect of your work experience would you recommend to a friend thinking about medicine, and why?
What would you do if you took a 'gap' year?
Can you think of a situation where good communication has saved the day and give a reason why?
How would you feel about writing about your volunteer work? (think about confidentiality.)

What experiences has your previous placement given you that will be useful in your medical career
Tell me about a patient you saw on work experience
What did you learn in G.P. surgery?
What role does everyone have in a team there
Tell me about your work experience
Why did you decide to do voluntary work? How did you come about it? What do you do there? What have you learnt?
Can you tell me the key things you learned from your work experience, in caring or other settings?
Reflecting on the work experience you have had in health or social care, can you identify some things you would like to change, and explain why?
What have you done on work experience/ in employment previously and what would you change about what you saw if you could?
What do you think would be the advantages, and difficulties, for a person with a major physical disability (e.g. blindness) wishing to become a doctor
Tell me about a project, or work experience, that you have organised,

and what you learned from it?

Is it a good idea to give aid to poor third world countries?
What do you think about involving the patient in their health care?
How do you think patients might best be involved in their health care?
In your career as a doctor you will probably look after people who are not going to get better. How do you think you would feel about this?
Why do you think it is that we cannot give a guarantee that a medical or surgical procedure will be successful?
What are the differences between length of life and quality of life?
Should alternative or complimentary medicine be funded by the NHS, and why?
How do you think doctors should address the issues of injury or illness due to smoking or drinking alcohol?
How will you cope with being criticised, or even perhaps being sued?
How do you think society should deal with beggars / any other marginalised group, and why?

Concerning motivation and realistic approach to medicine as a career:

What have you done to find out about medicine as a career/Who have you talked to about doing medicine and what did you learn from them?
What do you think you might like best about medicine as a career?
What do you feel are likely to be the worst things about being a doctor
When you visited a hospital, what did you see that set you thinking about the difficult aspects of a medical career?
What skills do you have that would make you a good doctor
What do you feel makes a good doctor
What difference did your work experience make to you?

Why medicine

Why are you suited to medicine
- What qualities would you regard as essential for a doctor

What qualities in a doctor are missing in you & do you think you can improve them

What makes a good team member & what have you noticed about working in a team

Have you ever been a leader, what does it involve

Give examples where you have used teamwork and leadership skills

Do you prefer being a team leader or a team worker

Give example of having to use communication skills in a tough situation

What experiences has your previous placement given you that will be useful in your medical career

Tell me about a patient you saw on work experience

How do you cope with stress

Do you read, what kind of books/newspapers

Tell us about the course

What diseases would you like to study with our resources

Limitations of PBL/self directed learning

Have you got any questions for us

Can you think of an example where doctors are faced with a difficult decision

What will you do if a person turns aggressive towards you

What would you do if a consultant shouted at you if you made a mistake

If a person while performing surgery attacked you what would you do

If there was an 80 year old woman in a critical condition and a 16 year old boy in a fairly stable but still critical condition who would you operate on first and why

What possible problems might you face as a consultant in 20 years

Pressures of being a doctor

How can being a G.P. be frustrating

Where do you see yourself in 10 years

What do you want to specialise in

Are there exams after university, what and with what board
Describe the path after medical school
What do GMC and RCS mean
What problems do the elderly encounter
How would you act around an elderly person you know if they found out they were terminally ill
What diseases should be resourced more

What changes in the last 50 years have affected the health or the nation
Talk about a medical/ethical issue that you've seen in the media that's caught your attention
(euthanasia, designer babies, cloning, religious issues e.g. Jehovah's witnesses & transfusion)
Bristol babies scandal was seen as a learning curve, what is your opinion
Have you heard about the human genome project
What recent medical breakthroughs have risen
Which medical documentaries have you seen recently
What do you know about MMR
Advances in medicine in the last 5/20/50/100 years
What was the most significant breakthrough in the last century
What do you think will be at the cutting edge of medicine in the next 20 years
Comment on the role of hospital management
Computer use in health care

Comment on teamwork and communication skills
What do you understand by the term good health
When was the NHS founded
How has the NHS revolutionised medicine
Who was the 1st NHS minister
Comment on the conflict between NHS and the government
• 4 things to mark the 50th anniversary of the NHS
Any dramatic changes since it was founded
Should we be made to pay for health care

Do you know how different the health system is in e.g. France
Comment on health care in developing countries
What do you think the NHS will be like in the future
If I gave you 10 million pounds for the NHS what would you do
Suggest how to reduce the costs of the NHS
If you were Alan Milburn what changes would you make to the NHS
What were the most recent NHS reforms
Consultants contract why did they turn down a 24% increase
What do you think about doctors private practice cut down
If you were prime minister what 3 government policies would you set to achieve
If you were to put together an ethical committee about genetic engineering who would you put on it
What are the key qualities a doctor should have?
Why is research important
- Do you think doctors make a difference to national health
What about the criticism of doctors nowadays
- What do you consider the main problems that confront doctors in training
What health problems are encountered in east London, general health of local population
What did you think of Body worlds & do you think Prof Van Hagen did autopsy for money
Who is your medical hero/who do you admire in the field of medicine
Do you think funding should be given to beggars and the homeless/ would you give money directly to beggars and why
What are you lacking and how would you develop these?
What are the major issues facing the NHS?
Is the NHS in crisis?
What are the major problems facing medicine?
What is the course system at Swansea?
What are your views on:
Genetic testing/insurance
Human cloning

Caesarean Operations

Are graduates better doctors than A level leavers?
What would you do if you didn't get into medicine?
Do you know what the course structure is?
What is PBL and the spiral curriculum?
Is it a good way to learn and teach?
What is the greatest discovery in the past 100 years?
What is the greatest advancement in the past 50 years?
Hippocratic oath?
Why medicine and not science (Was a medical physicist before)?

Contribution to Medical School life:and the personal statement

Which activities do you think you would like to do?
Would you like to do something new or continue your music/drama/mountaineering (or similar)?
What would you like people to remember about you from your medical school life?
The medical course is hard work. How do you propose to manage your work and still play football/violin (or similar)?
Questions relating to the personal statement

General tips on the interview

Read newspapers in the months before your interview
Try and get hold of a journal from a library/parent BMJ/NEJM/New Scientist
Read through your CV/statement so you know what you have written
Look at your personal statement with an eye for potential questions.
Why medicine, this university
Admit if you don't know an answer
Say if you need time to think
Practice with friends/relatives
They are more interested in the way you frame your answer than the

answer itself.
For ethical dilemmas they want to see that you are able to see issues from other peoples perspective.
Remember body language, smile, be confident, lean forward
Thank the interviewers

Positive behavioural indicators

The following indicators are now used in the selection of general practitioners and are being expanded for the selection of other specialities and almost certainly will make up the indicators looked for in aptitude tests and interviews. In the G.P. selection process an examiner records comments made by the interviewee and then assesses how these compare with the marking scheme below.

Empathy/sensitivity; open, non judgemental, cooperative, warmth and encouragement
Communication skills; express ideas clearly, effective non verbal behaviour, humour, analogy
Problem solving; think around the issue, open to possibilities, generate functional solution, timekeeping, identify key issues
Integrity; respect, enthusiastic, positive, admit mistakes, equality, back own judgement appropriately
Coping with pressure; calm, don't lose sight of wider needs, recognise own limitations, compromise, seek help, strategies to deal with stress

Chapter 4

Possible answers to common questions

Possible Interview Questions Answered

I have attempted to answer the following questions providing up to date information at the same time. You may well be able to answer them in a more original way. Try not to be too formulaic and if you have an interesting new slant on a question do not hesitate to use it, it might make you stand out from the crowd.

Why have you chosen to do medicine?	199
What interests you about medicine?	199
What are your limitations or weaknesses	200
Do you have any career intentions?	200
Why not be a nurse if you want to help people?	200
Tell me about an article you have read in a newspaper or journal recently that relates to medicine	200
Tell me about NHS policies such as 'choose and book', 'payment by results', practice based commissioning, MMC	201
What groups would you imagine working with in your role as a doctor	202
Who do you think is the most important member of a multi disciplinary health care team? Why?	201
What are the advantages and disadvantages of being in a team?	203
Are you a leader or a team player	203

How do you cope with stress	203
Can you think of an example where doctors are faced with a difficult decision	202
What would you do if a consultant shouted at you if you made a mistake	203
Tell me about a patient you saw on your work experience? Why did this person stand out in your mind?	203
What aspect of your work experience did you find the most and least interesting, and why?	204
In your work experience, what skills have you learnt that you can apply to medicine?	204
Reflect on what you have seen of hospitals or a health care environment. What would you most like to organise differently, and why?	204
What aspect of your work experience would you recommend to a friend thinking about medicine, and why?	204
Is it a good idea to give aid to poor third world countries?	205
What do you think about involving the patient in their health care?	206
How do you think patients might best be involved in their health care?	206
Why do you think it is that we cannot give a guarantee that a medical or surgical procedure will be successful?	206
What are the differences between length of life and quality	207

of life?

In your career as a doctor you will probably look after people who are not going to get better. How do you think you would feel about this?	211
How will you cope with being criticised, or even perhaps being sued?	211
How do you think society should deal with beggars or other marginalised group, and why?	212
Should alternative or complimentary medicine be funded by the NHS, and why?	212
What do you understand by problem based learning (PBL)?	212
What are the limitations of PBL/self directed learning	213
Tell us about the course	213
What diseases would you like to study with our resources	213
Who do you register with after your foundation year? What is the foundation programme? What does MMC mean? What do GMC and RCS mean.	213
Where do you see yourself in 10 years	215
What are the arguments for and against nonessential surgery being available on the NHS?	215

Why do you think an NHS Trust has recently proposed to limit the access of very obese patients to certain types of surgery? Can you think of any arguments

for / against this?	217
What does the current government see as the national priorities in health care? Do you agree with these?	219
What changes in the last 50 years have helped the health of the nation?	219
Have you heard about the human genome project	219
What do you know of the MMR vaccine	222
What recent medical breakthroughs have arisen	223
Which medical documentaries have you seen recently?	223
What skills do you think are needed in order to communicate with your patients; how do you think they are best acquired?	224
How would you like your patients to describe you	225
What interests do you bring from school/college life that you think will contribute to your studies and practice?	225
Have there been any particular life experiences that you think will help you in a career in medicine?	226
What challenges do you think a career in medicine will bring you?	226
What do you think you will be the most negative aspects of being a doctor	226

What do you think you will be the most positive aspects of being a doctor	226
What attributes are necessary in a good doctor	226
The duties of a doctor registered with the General Medical Council	226
Which activities do you think you would like to do? Would you like to do something new or continue your music/drama/mountaineering?	227
What would you like people to remember about you from your medical school life?	227
The medical course is hard work. How do you propose to manage your work and still play football/violin?	227
Suggest how to reduce the costs of the NHS	227
If you were Alan Milburn what changes would you make to the NHS	227
Should we be made to pay for health care	228
Do you know how different the health system is in e.g. France	228
Comment on health care in developing countries	228
What do you think the NHS will be like in the future	228
If I gave you 10 million pounds for the NHS what would you do	228
What were the most recent NHS reforms	229

Consultants contract why did they turn down a 24% increase

What do you think about doctor's private practice being reduced?	229
Ethical scenarios	229
Which is more important general practice (primary care) or hospital, and why?	230
Do you think euthanasia should be legalised? Discuss the pros and cons. Should life be prolonged at all costs?	230
Do you think the country needs more doctors or more nurses? What do you think will be the effects of having more female doctors than male doctors?	233
What are the arguments for and against banning the sale of tobacco?	234
Why do doctors sometimes get a bad press?	235
What is meant by the inequalities of health and what can be done to reduce them?	236
As a doctor, you have killed someone who otherwise would have survived how would you deal with that? What do you tell family	236
A patient comes to you with a newspaper clipping suggesting that a new drug might be better than the one he takes. It is three times the cost to prescribe. What are the ethical issues raised.	237
Are you aware of any changes to the cervical	237

screening program?	
What are your views on genetic testing and insurance?	237
Everyone knows that doctors treat ill people. What else do you think doctors do?	238
What health problems are encountered in East London. Is the NHS in crisis?	238
When was the NHS formed, who was the first minister for the NHS	239
Why do we need screening and how do we carry it out.	241
Are there exams after university, what are they? Describe the path after medical school	242
What do you think of nurses developing extended roles and undertaking tasks previously done by doctors?	244
What do you think about the proposal that nurses could replace doctors as the first contact person in primary care?	244
Tell us what attracts you most and least about this Medical School	244
"You are the head of panel for the proposition of changing every London taxi to vehicles with Hybrid engines. What would you include in your report?	244
What is The path after Medical school and what are the arguments for and against MMC?	245
What is confidentiality? When can a doctor breach	249

confidentiality?

How would you cope with a difficult patient? What types are there?	256
What one question would you ask if interviewing others interested in studying medicine?	260
What are the health implications of global warming?	070
What are the pros and cons of cloning?	260
How do you think the rise in information technology has influenced and will influence the practice of medicine?	268
Ten years ago most doctors in hospitals wore white coats; now few do. Why do you think this is? What do you think are the arguments for and against white coats?	269
What problems do you think the widespread use of recreational drugs pose to doctors?	269
Female infertility treatment is expensive, has a very low success rate and is even less successful in smokers. To whom do you think it should be available?	270
Can you give me an example of how you coped with a conflict with a colleague or friend; what strategy did you use and why?	270
Have you ever been in a situation where you realise afterwards that what you said or did was wrong? What did you do about it? What should you have done?	272
Give us an example of something about which you used to hold strong opinions, but have had to change your mind.	272

What made you change? What do you think now?

What is your opinion on "Widening access to Medicine courses?" 273

What happens between the time a pharmacist invents a drug and a doctor prescribing it. 273

What are the pros and cons of pharmaceutical representatives visiting doctors to promote their drugs? 273

Possible answers to common questions

Why have you chosen to do medicine?

Make your reasons as specific as possible. Use anecdotes of what experiences made you decide to do medicine, it might have been as the result of a childhood trip to hospital. You can also acknowledge the 'down side' to the job such as the hours, responsibilities, expectation of patients. This makes the interviewer aware that you have thought about the career you have chosen. State what you have done to get better informed, it might be work experience, reading about the NHS or talking to doctors.

You might want to mention that you have attended a premed course and what you learned from the experience.
Examiners dislike clichés such as 'I want to help people or make the world a better place. One interviewee was asked if she regretted a particularly sugary opening line to her personal statement!

You might want to think about how science interfaces with art and the humanities. A common question might be 'how does your classic civilisation course help with a possible career in medicine?'

What interests you about medicine?

Again, be specific and anecdotal. You can mention a specific patient/clinical situation and what caught your imagination. If you can, invoke an inspiring doctor you have known, say why he or she inspired you, avoid being overly gushing though. You can mention medical article you have read, indeed you should have one in mind as candidates are frequently asked about a recent medicine related story they might have read about.

Again mention the challenges as well as positives and be able to answer when they ask how you might deal with these challenges. Avoid kudos and salary as reasons to enter medicine.

What are your limitations or weaknesses?

The best solution is to choose answers that are not really weaknesses. For example, you might say that you're rather a perfectionist. Explain that this could be a limitation when you go to university because with the busy schedule of being a medicine student and a doctor it will be difficult to do things to your high standards, but that you will have to work on this during the course. Avoid saying things such as I am easily stressed or depressed or that you are not a great communicator or have problems mixing.

You could say that you are prone to get too involved in your work or have not quite got your work/life balance right at present but that you recognise this. Avoid 'I work too hard'

You might say, 'I can get impatient when I can see a solution to a problem but am not quite sure how to reach that point'.
Show that you have been thought about what you learned about yourself, about he needs of patients and about the teams you have experienced during your work experience.

Do you have any career intentions?

There is no reason to expect you to have developed a confirmed interest in any one field of medicine. It is reasonable to suggest that you have little experience of many fields of medicine. You might say though I am particularly interested in being a surgeon because I am dextrous and enjoy the technical aspect of surgery and the fact that one can offer a complete solution to a problem with a single operation'.

Your answer here must go beyond 'I am particularly interested in dermatology/psychiatry…' , you should explain why you have an interest that goes beyond 'its the only speciality I have experience of. Invoke specific experiences within the speciality if you have any.

Don't be too rigid about choices – admit that you don't know enough yet to make an informed choice.

Why not be a nurse if you want to help people?

This question illustrates why you should avoid stating that you wish to help people!

Do not criticise nurses, instead praise their role as essential.

Your training as a doctor will give you a much more in depth understanding of disease and its management. Your training will be broader and will allow you greater freedom in prescribing than for instance nurse practitioners that can prescribe but in limited, protocol driven situations. Doctors have ultimate responsibility for patient care and tend to be the decision makers. Medicine is likely to be more intellectually challenging and will offer more possibilities for research. The variety of career opportunities is very broad from an academic role to a hands on consultant, a G.P. who gains a broader understanding of different fields of medicine, occupational health doctors, legal advisers, sports medicine specialists.

Tell me about an article you have read in a newspaper or journal recently that relates to medicine

You really must in the months leading up to your interview, scan the papers for interesting stories. Probably the Daily Mail is the most medicine obsessed paper. If you have a relative who takes a medical journal, by all means read that but avoid complex articles that you will not understand and be able to explain clearly. The issues change from time to time. Obesity seems here to stay and is taxing the government with regard to the long term health time bomb it represents. Rationing is a perennial issue and you should know of a drug such as herceptin that is expensive and is causing difficulties with funding.

Issues around the human genome and how the discovery of the genome might lead to breakthroughs in treatment of certain disease such as cancers and single gene diseases such as cystic fibrosis. Stem cell research is very topical. Stem cells are the earliest cells produced and they have the capacity to transform into any mature cell type such as a muscle cell, red cell or brain cell. This offers the possibility of treating the stem cell in such a way that it divides to produce the type of cell you are seeking, perhaps heart muscle cells to heal a heart damaged by a heart attack.

Tell me about NHS policies such as 'choose and book', 'payment by results' , practice based commissioning, MMC

Choose and book is an IT system that links G.P.s to hospital providers allowing instant booking of appointments so that patients can choose a convenient time. It is also linked to the government's choice agenda whereby primary care trusts must offer a number of choices to patients including independent sector or private providers.
'Payment by results' refers to the process whereby hospitals get paid for their activity. For example, if a patient is admitted to hospital for removal of their appendix the hospital will get paid a 'tariff' price for the procedure. Tariff prices are mapped out for all possible eventualities be it a hip replacement or sinus operation.
Practice based commissioning is a process whereby G.P.s are given the commissioning budget, that is the budget from which all procedures are paid, and are able to decide how it is aspect. This has led to G.P.s providing services in different ways. Perhaps running a diabetes clinic from the surgery instead of from the hospital outpatient department so reducing the cost.
MMC is modernising medical careers, a radical change in the career structure for training doctors. The career pathway now starts with the 'foundation programme' the first two years of postgraduate training for all doctors. This consists of six four month attachments to specialities including general practice. After the foundation programme, doctors apply to join higher specialist training schemes that can last for anything from 3 years to 7 years depending upon the

speciality. MMC is designed to match supply of doctors trained to the number of vacancies available.

The EWD European working time directive states the number of hours a doctor can work in an average week and this has lead to a change in the way doctors work. The hours are reduced but the work load is more intense whilst they are working as they must cover a wider area of the hospital to allow for the reduced number of doctors working at any one time.

What groups would you imagine working with in your role as a doctor

As a doctor you are ultimately likely to be a team leader whether it be running a General practice or a hospital department. You will though need to work with a diverse group of people, technicians, nurses, porters, theatre assistants.. It is therefore, important to show you can work with a team. Express the important features of a team player; good communications skills with the ability to both express ideas and listen to those of others, supportive and non judgmental, reliability, flexibility.

Who do you think is the most important member of a multi disciplinary health care team? Why?

The most important member of a team is its leader, poor leadership is likely to result in dysfunction. You might also say that the team is limited by its weakest link so it is important to get everyone on board and ensure that appropriate people are appointed to positions within the team.

What are the advantages and disadvantages of being in a team?

The disadvantage of working in a team might be that if you work as an individual you can have more freedom to express new ideas, lack of leadership can make a team dysfunctional, the more team members there are, the less likely a decision will be made. The advantages include support, opportunities to learn from other specialists, social aspects of teamwork.

Are you a leader or a team player

There are several similarities between a team leader and a team player and you might wish to point this out when asked. For instance, the ability to communicate, work with a team, be supportive and non judgmental. Where they differ is the ability to take decisions, meld a team together, set objectives and be approachable and command respect. You should have some examples available where you showed leadership or worked within a team.

How do you cope with stress

This question will probably appear in one guise or another, medicine can be stressful at times as can your period as a medical student facing a high workload combined with new experiences of illness and death.
In coping with stress you should show evidence of remaining calm, delegating work where it is reasonable to do so, seeking help and support from other team members, developing coping strategies such as exercise or yoga, developing your time management skills so that you do not put excessive pressure upon yourself. Take breaks from a stressful situation if possible and where possible confront an issue such as a difficult colleague

Can you think of an example where doctors are faced with a difficult decision

Typical difficult decisions might be lack of resources causing you to ration or offer a treatment that is inferior due to lack of funding. When to switch off a life support machine, which of three acute

emergencies to tackle first.
If attacked there are issues around protecting yourself, your staff and the patient Call for help, try to remain calm, do not raise your voice, try to reason with the patient, protect yourself and your staff as best you can

What would you do if a consultant shouted at you if you made a mistake

If shouted at by a consultant, try to remain calm, explain that you are a medical student and do not expect your seniors to behave in this way. Advise the consultant that because you are a student you have much to learn and that you are sorry of that has angered them and that you will endeavour to learn by your mistakes. If the attack was personal or racially motivated, if you have a tutor or mentor assigned to you report the incident to them, if not advise them that you will be forced to report to the Director of the department
With regard to coping with pressure, the positive indicators looked for in a doctor are as follows;

Coping with pressure; calm, don't lose sight of wider needs, recognise own limitations, compromise, seek help, strategies to deal with stress.

Positive indicators are basically buzz words that describe the behavioural traits being looked for in a given scenario. When you answer a question on stress bare them in mind and try and choose a scenario or reply that illustrates these traits.

Tell me about a patient you saw on your work experience? Why did this person stand out in your mind?

You need to select a patient that stood out for a reason you can relate. Do not select someone who stood out on the basis of the amount of vomit they could produce in a day. Good choices might include someone who stood out because of bravery or stoicism, someone who changed your opinion on the mentally handicapped or disabled, perhaps someone who had an interesting disease or procedure. Say something about yourself rather than the other doctors or staff. How did it make you feel, what did you learn about yourself or the world?

What aspect of your work experience did you find the most and least interesting, and why?

If you mention something that did not interest you be prepared to explain why. You might say that the diagnostic challenge of neurology interested me whereas surgery is a practical task that would not be suited to my skills as I lack the degree of dexterity that I am sure would be required to perform the job well.

In your work experience, what skills have you learnt that you can apply to medicine?

It is important that you find work experience. It need not be in a hospital or G.P. surgery, find work with the disabled, mentally handicapped, demented, elderly, in a shop or portering. These all improve communication skills and involve dealing with people who have one difficulty or another. Skills that you might learn are communication skills, negotiation, an awareness of some of the problems your clients face, organisational and time management skills. Listening skills, handling difficult people, perhaps leadership opportunities, explaining complex problems in a simple way are all skills that can be transferred to medicine so mention a few of them when asked.

Reflect on what you have seen of hospitals or a health care environment. What would you most like to organise differently, and why?

Think before the interview of something that happened that you particularly enjoyed. Be specific, explain the situation, do not fabricate, you will be spotted, personalise it rather than talk about what others did. Explain what happened and why and what the outcome of the event was. If you are going to describe something bad, try and avoid criticism of individuals. Rather perhaps say, some of the clinics ran very late, this seemed to be because only one nurse was available for two doctors and this led to delays whilst they waited for a chaperone. If a second nurse or trained chaperone was used at relatively low cost the doctors would have been more productive.

What aspect of your work experience would you recommend to a friend thinking about medicine, and why?

What did you most enjoy and why? Again they are not looking for the actions of others but rather 'what did you do in the scenario. Perhaps, choose something in which you were allowed to participate, it need not be medical, just interesting.

Attitudinal questions

With these questions, interviewers are looking at attitude, empathy and evidence that you have shown some interest in the world around you.

Is it a good idea to give aid to poor third world countries?

Think broadly, comment on how the situation affects the doctor, the patient, the hospital and the wider society.
Giving aid to the third world might have advantages and disadvantages. It is important how aid is spent, if used on sustainable projects it helps a community rebuild itself, if used to continually supply food for instance, it might induce a dependant culture in a society that prides itself on independence and just needs a helping hand perhaps to provide new seed grain for the next harvest because the previous harvest failed. Flooding a third world market with certain items may put local merchants out of business and ultimately worsen the situation.

<u>What do you think about involving the patient in their health care?</u>
<u>How do you think patients might best be involved in their health care?</u>

With regard to patient involvement in health care, mention autonomy, the right of a patient to be fully informed and involved in decision making when it comes to their own health. Discuss doctor-patient partnership groups who get together to feed back to the doctor Mention support groups such as the multiple sclerosis society that provide up to date information and support to sufferers. Talk about patient education through the media or through family doctors, which empowers patients.

<u>Why do you think it is that we cannot give a guarantee that a medical or surgical procedure will be successful?</u>

There can be no guarantees when it comes to treatment. It may be unsuccessful or even harmful. This raises the question of informed consent. It is important that a patient is fully informed of the potential benefits, risks of a procedure and the likelihood of success. In order to do this a patient must be deemed competent. Competence refers to the ability of a patient to understand the information they are being given, it comprises the ability to comprehend information, believe it and weigh up the information to make a decision. A competent adult can refuse even life saving treatment. Treatment may be unsuccessful due to differences in the way patients react to the treatment for example some patients have an abnormal liver enzyme system that makes them handle drugs in a different way. There may be differences in the way a disease responds to treatment in different patients. Cancers may be more aggressive in some than others, organisms may be resistant to antibiotics.

<u>What are the differences between length of life and quality</u>

of life?

Length of life is self explanatory, quality of life is harder to measure but QALY or quality of life years is a measure adopted to look at the benefits of certain treatments over an alternative treatment.

MicroAllocation vs MacroAllocation
- Microlevel allocation involves making decisions about which specific patient is to receive an available treatment
- Macro allocation involves decisions at a higher level. These decisions range from whether a clinical department ought to invest in a new piece of equipment, to broad questions about the health services to be provided by a health care system.

Age is an allocation criterion that can be applied in a number of ways. It has even been suggested that, in some allocation situations, older people have a duty to forgo treatment in favour of younger candidates.

Responsibility for Disease: if a person needing treatment is responsible for her illness, some would suggest that this ought to reduce her priority. Two key issues arise from these considerations. Is it right to reduce priority on grounds of responsibility for disease? We allow people to come to harm as a result of their own decisions in many areas of life (e.g. financial planning), but should health care be different?
To what degree may we say a person is responsible for his or her illness? Behaviour may be the result of a depressive illness, related to genetic factors or upbringing.
Prognosis: how successful treatment is likely to be is another factor to be considered. Criteria of success include improved quality and quantity of life. The QALY approach gives major weight to these considerations.

Length of Time Waiting: we might take into account the length of time the patient has been waiting for treatment. It can be a factor in decisions about allocation within the NHS, in the form of waiting lists – a patient's place on the list has a role, with other factors, in determining when treatment will be allocated.

Benefit to Others: the benefits to society of an intervention can sometimes have a role. Dependent children and continuing business activities will be of benefit to society.

Desert: considerations rely on judgements of the worth or merit of a person.

Ability to Pay: one of the cornerstones of the NHS is that health care ought to be allocated on the basis of clinical need rather than ability to pay. However, those who can afford private medicine are often able to purchase better health care than those who cannot. Such inequities in health care are even more marked in health care systems that lack a well funded public sector.

Urgency of Need: is the criterion that is likely to have the most significant role.

QALYs
One promising solution to the problem would be to focus on the cost effectiveness of treatment. The QALY is a tool designed to do this.
Calculation of the QALY involves an assessment of quality of life and its relationship to illness. This quality assessment is multiplied by the number of years for which the quality of life will be maintained. For example, suppose coronary artery bypass surgery raises a person's quality of life form 0.6 to 0.9, an increase of 0.3. If the surgery maintains this increase for 10 years, and if this person would have lived at 0.6 for 10 years without the surgery, the surgery can be said to produce 3 QALYs (0.3x10 years).
The possibility of a negative quality of life is important in QALY theory. Some medical treatments (e.g. for severe burns) have recovery periods during which (arguably) the patient's quality of

life is worse than being dead. In such situations, the first QALYs produced may be negative.

Measuring cost effectiveness requires a consideration of how much effectiveness costs. This can be achieved relatively simply using QALYs.

Using the QALY approach, 1 year of healthy life expectancy is worth 1 and 1 year of unhealthy life is worth <1. The lower the QALY value, the worse the quality of life. If being dead is worth zero, it is, in principle, possible for a QALY to be negative – the quality of the person's life is judged worse than being dead.

Because QALYs focus on the cost effectiveness of treatments, they do not take account of responsibility for illness, length of waiting time, benefit to others, desert, ability to pay or urgency of need. Supporters of the QALY approach disagree whether it ought to be used for micro allocation decisions.

Ageism
Younger people have longer to live, so have an 'unfair' advantage in QALY calculations. The QALY approach is likely to favour relatively more funding for paediatrics and less for gerontology, and this fact has prompted Harris and other critics to claim that QALYs are inherently ageist. Others argue that QALYs are not ageist enough. According to the QALY approach, an 80 year old with a life expectancy of 5 years would be dealt with in the same way as a 40 year old with a life expectancy of 5 years.

Double Jeopardy
Using QALYs, people whose quality of life is already low may be given lower priority treatment than those with a high quality of life. Consider the case of two people, one with severe arthritis, both of whom need life extending treatment for a reason unrelated to arthritis (e.g. cardiac problems). Both would receive the same life extension at the same cost. However, the cost per QALY would be greater for the person with arthritis because his quality of life is

lower. Using the QALY approach, he would be given lower priority for cardiac treatment.

Alternative medicine may have its part to play in medicine, chiropraxy, osteopathy, aromatherapy, accupuncture and reflexology were all perceived as black magic by doctors 25 years ago. They have largely entered the main stream, particularly in cancer therapy. You need to be able to discuss the lack of an evidence base for many therapies. Talk about the limitation of funding in the NHS and the need to target funds on evidence based treatments, that is treatments that have been shown to work in controlled trials. Mention the widespread use of accupuncture for chronic pain control in NHS pain clinics.

In your career as a doctor you will probably look after people who are not going to get better. How do you think you would feel about this?

With regard to patients who do not get better, point out that one can gain great satisfaction from palliating disease, that is relieving symptoms in someone that is dying of cancer, lung disease or heart failure. Recognise there will be times when the loss of a patient will have a considerable impact on you and talk about how talking to friends and colleagues can help with such cases. You also have to recognise that modern medicine has made great strides but that everyone will still die of something and that you cannot expect to treat everyone successfully.

How will you cope with being criticised, or even perhaps being sued?

Coping with complaints or being sued is difficult for anyone to deal with. It is a criticism of your care and your ability. You will need to remain calm, analyse the case, look at it either alone or with a mentor to determine how you might have dealt with the case differently. If you have been at fault, make an early appointment with the complainant to apologise and explain what went wrong and which steps you have taken to prevent it happening again.

How do you think society should deal with beggars / any other marginalised group, and why?

In dealing with marginalised groups such as beggars, you need first to understand why they have arrived at the current situation. If it the result of alcoholism or mental health issues then it makes sense to address these problems, similarly, if they have drug problems then encouraging them to seek rehabilitation would be appropriate. You need to recognise the difficulties they might have in accessing help such as travel issues and the lack of a fixed abode. You might wish to set up a hostel or a back to work scheme that will allow such people to re enter the work force in a controlled way and with appropriate training. They will have particular health issues such as infections like tuberculosis, liver disease resulting from alcohol abuse or HIV resulting from using dirty needles.

Should alternative or complimentary medicine be funded by the NHS, and why?

Review the evidence. There is little evidence for many alternative therapies. Some that were once considered 'quack' medicine have become mainstream. Aromatherapists and reflexologists and accupuncturists are used by cancer clinics and pain clinics. Patients feel better after the former and there is some evidence that accupuncture is useful for chronic pain. There are homeopathy hospital in the UK, homeopathy is based, I believe on the notion that you give a patient a diluted version of a substance that would cause the symptoms they are complaining of. The more diluted, the more powerful. There is little research evidence for homeopathy working but its use is widespread. There are arguments that there is a strong placebo effect due to the fact that patients are listened to for long periods. As to whether it should be provided on the NHS, you should argue that only evidence based medicine should be available on the NHS. Mention the issue of justice, autonomy, non-malifisense.

What do you understand by problem based learning (PBL)?

PBL is problem based learning a new style of learning adopted by several medical schools. Put simply, it means teaching using a problem as the starting point. For example, lung cancer would provide a starting point from which students would learn the basic anatomy, physiology and treatment of lung cancer, rather than the more typical method of learning anatomy and physiology in the first two years and clinical work for the remaining 3 years.

What are the limitations of PBL/self directed learning

This form of learning is a more mature form of learning which requires motivation and the ability to go off and seek answers for yourself, rather than being presented with a lecture. It is easier with PBL to get patchy coverage of a subject. For instance, you might cover lung cancer and chronic obstructive pulmonary disease but may not cover a whole range of other lung diseases that might be more fully covered by a lecture with handout notes. The advantages though are that the anatomy and physiology become much more interesting when you are dealing with a real patient with a real disease.

Tell us about the course

This illustrates the importance of reading the prospectus and establishing the type of course being run. Is it traditional or is it problem based or a mix of the two. Is there an intercalated BSc, a further degree taken over a year, usually after year 3 or 4, some universities offer this as an option, others insist you take one.

What diseases would you like to study with our resources

If you choose a disease you will need to explain why you feel it is important. Choose either a major killer such as cancer, a disease which has a high morbidity such as diabetes or one to which you have a strong attachment, perhaps a family member suffers from it.

Who do you register with after your foundation year? What is the foundation programme? What does MMC mean? What do GMC and RCS mean.

You register with the General Medical Council (GMC) the body that oversees behaviour among doctors and has the power to remove you from the register should you break the moral code.
The foundation programme is a new two year programme of six four month posts or jobs. It replaced a one year pre-registration house job and a year as a senior house officer. After these six varied jobs which ideally include the job or jobs you hope to continue with, you enter a specialist training or ST programme. In General Practice this is three years, other specialities may be 5 years.

MMC or Modernising Medical Careers is described thus on the MMC web site 'Modernising Medical Careers (MMC) aims to improve patient care by delivering a modernised and focused career structure for doctors through a major reform of postgraduate medical education. It aims to develop demonstrably competent doctors who are skilled at communicating and working as effective members of a team. As training and education are central to the work of doctors and their role in delivering patient care, MMC will also bring about significant changes to career structures, providing qualified staff who are able to meet the needs of patients.

To do this, MMC has created two year foundation schools that will, for the first time, require doctors to demonstrate their abilities and competence against set standards. There will be an opportunity to develop experience in a range of specialities. This will offer doctors the chance to gain insight into possible career options or to build a wider appreciation of medicine before embarking on specialist training.

Postfoundation, specialist/G.P. training will be streamlined to deliver specialists who are judgement safe and able to deliver the care that is needed to treat patients, without compromising in any way on standards. Streamlined training will also afford further opportunities for super specialisation that are flexible enough to allow doctors to adapt to accommodate changes in medical technology. In this way the new system under MMC aims to provide the right numbers of doctors to meet changing service needs.

Streamlined training and explicit standards of assessed competence are also essential if doctors' careers are to accommodate the pressures of a family and modern lifestyles. MMC aims to greatly improve the opportunities for those who wish to take a break in their careers and will promote fairness and equality of opportunity at all stages of a doctors' career.

RCS is the Royal College of Surgeons, there are royal colleges for all of the specialities and they monitor training and plan how careers in a given speciality will develop in the future. RCP RC of Physicians, RCOG, RC of obstetricians and Gynaecologists etc.

Where do you see yourself in 10 years

This can be tricky if you do not think ahead of the interview. This is a chance to give a broad brush answer about yourself. You will have developed a number of skills in your medical training, particularly communications skills, specific technical skills, time keeping , organisational, team working and leadership skills. You will hopefully have developed your extracurricular interests, sports, music the arts. You may well have a family. Your interest in medicine/surgery/paediatrics (delete as appropriate) suggests that you may well have a career in that subject but you appreciate that you will have a better perspective on this as time passes. You are likely to want to develop your teaching skills .

What are the arguments for and against nonessential surgery being available on the NHS?

One needs to establish the meaning of the word nonessential. Breast reduction or augmentation might be considered a cosmetic procedure but I can think of two patients in whom it had significant medical benefits. One had such large breasts that she had significant back problems and one had had a sex change procedure and was suicidally depressed at the fact her breasts had failed to develop.
Failure to fund procedures may push patients to over stretching their finances or to go abroad to less regulated health providers for cheaper surgery. One might also argue that when the NHS was developed it was advertised as a 'cradle to grave' heath service that would deal with all your health needs.
Against nonessential surgery are the arguments that health provision is a bottomless pit and that because essential surgery cannot be controlled, the only element of control is over nonessential procedures.
Rationing can be either explicit, that is driven by protocol or NICE guidance or implicit, rationing by waiting list, prejudice or tradition. With regard to limiting treatment in people who smoke, drank or eat too much, the GMC guidance is that it is unethical to withhold treatment on the basis of lifestyle.
With regard to deciding whom to treat if two equally deserving patients need an ITU bed or expensive treatment, you could argue that doctors are not best placed to make these decisions and that a study on the use of ITU beds showed that clinical suitability and potential benefit did not determine who got beds but rather political power of the doctors involved and income maximisation.

If asked such a question fall back upon the theories of justice

Utilitarian
Striving to provide the maximum health benefit for the greatest number of patients.

Libertarian
There is no right to health care but rather it is a choice that can be paid for, this benefits the rich and neglects the poor.

Communitarian
This is counter to the libertarian argument and suggests that health care should be distributed on the basis of needs and goals. How these are defined is determined by society.

Egalitarian
The main aim here is to provide an environment where all can achieve equally. Health care is merely a means whereby people are not prevented from this goal by illness

Why do you think an NHS Trust has recently proposed to limit the access of very obese patients to certain types of surgery? Can you think of any arguments for / against this?]

Arguments for by Doctor Jonathan Fielden, chairman of the British Medical Association's consultants' committee in the Daily Telegraph 30/01/07

Although politicians are loath to admit it, there has always been some form of rationing in the NHS, whether in the form of waiting lists, or treatments being ruled out because the clinical case for them is insufficiently strong. Cosmetic surgery, for example, is rarely carried out on the NHS. We strongly believe in an NHS free at the point of delivery and funded from general taxation. However from 2008, the year on year funding increases that the NHS has seen in recent years will drop significantly.

Meanwhile, the population is ageing and expectations are rising. Hospitals are dealing with increasing volumes of patients, and the costs of drugs and new technologies continue to rise. NHS trusts are in deficit during this time of feast, let alone the coming famine.

The public should be trusted to debate what a comprehensive health service is and how much they are willing to pay. The result must be universal and equitable or the ethos of the NHS will be lost.

While this discussion needs to be professionally led, politicians must be honest about what funds are available, and the public must be allowed a real say. However, the debate on where NHS money goes should be about more than which treatments are available – it should also focus on who provides them.

While the NHS may be unable to meet all demand for services, it has historically provided excellent value for money — a claim that cannot be made about all the private firms currently profiting from the NHS.

Argument against by Professor John Appleby, chief economist at the King's Fund

Doomsday predictions about the inability of the NHS to cope with demand pressures have been made for decades — yet the NHS continues to cope.

Clearly, there is only so much money the NHS has to spend each year and decisions have to be made about what it spends its money on — crudely, who gets what and when. This has always been true and will remain so despite new costly drugs coming along.

The NHS is facing one of its most challenging periods. But there is nothing particularly special about the next few years that will reduce the NHS — as some claim — to a rump of a service, only able to provide a mere basic level of care.

We used to think that an ageing population would eventually lead to the NHS going bust, but as of yet this hasn't happened, although pressures on the health service from rising numbers of older people will increase over the next 20 years.

And there are always those who say that new, expensive drugs will mean that the NHS will find it difficult to afford everything that is medically possible. But again, this has always been the case. But further, many of the new cancer drugs, for example, are not just costly, but have marginal impacts on health. In other words, there will be serious doubt about whether they will be "good buys" for the NHS.

The debate about NHS rationing is not whether it should be done, but how it should be done given that as a society we have taken the decision not to ration access to health care on the basis of price and the individual's ability to pay.

What does the current government see as the national priorities in health care? Do you agree with these?

The Choosing health White Paper includes

- Radical action to increase the number of smoke free work places
- Curbs on the promotion of unhealthy foods to children
- Clear, unambiguous labelling of the nutritional content of food
- NHS Health Trainers to provide advice to individuals on how to improve their lifestyle
- A wide range of measures to tackle social and geographical inequalities in health

The governments current national priorities also include reducing obesity, improving mental health provision, sexual health, and improving cancer survival.

What changes in the last 50 years have helped the health of the nation?

Do not forget to mention improved housing and nutrition. Antibiotics arrived in the 1940s but have been developed considerably in the last 50 years. Imaging has been a major breakthrough, we can now have a much clearer picture of what is going on inside a person through MRI and CT without the need to operate. Safer anaesthetics have played a major part in making surgery safer. Changes in practice such as shorter hospital stays due to 'keyhole' surgery have reduced the complications of surgery such as blood clots.

Have you heard about the human genome project

The human genome project

Project goals were to

Identify all the approximately genes in human DNA,
Determine the sequences of the 3 billion chemical base pairs that make up human DNA,
Store this information in databases,
improve tools for data analysis,
transfer related technologies to the private sector, and
address the ethical, legal, and social issues (ELSI) that may arise from the project.

Benefits according to the web site (http://www.ornl.gov/sci/techresources/Human_Genome/home.shtml) include;

Molecular Medicine
Improved diagnosis of disease
Earlier detection of genetic predisposition's to disease
Rational drug design
Gene therapy and control systems for drugs
Pharmacogenomics "custom drugs

Energy and Environmental Applications
Use microbial genomics research to create new energy sources (biofuels)

Use microbial genomics research to develop environmental monitoring techniques to detect pollutants
Use microbial genomics research for safe, efficient environmental remediation
Use microbial genomics research for carbon sequestration

Risk Assessment
Assess health damage and risks caused by radiation exposure, including low dose exposures
Assess health damage and risks caused by exposure to mutagenic chemicals and cancer causing toxins
Reduce the likelihood of heritable mutations

Bioarchaeology, Anthropology, Evolution, and Human Migration

Study evolution through germline mutations in lineages
Study migration of different population groups based on female genetic inheritance
Study mutations on the Y chromosome to trace lineage and migration of males
Compare breakpoints in the evolution of mutations with ages of populations and historical events

DNA Forensics (Identification)

Identify potential suspects whose DNA may match evidence left at crime scenes
Exonerate persons wrongly accused of crimes
Identify crime and catastrophe victims
Establish paternity and other family relationships
Identify endangered and protected species as an aid to wildlife officials (could be used for prosecuting poachers)
Detect bacteria and other organisms that may pollute air, water, soil, and food
Match organ donors with recipients in transplant programs
Determine pedigree for seed or livestock breeds

Authenticate consumables such as caviar and wine

Agriculture, Livestock Breeding, and Bioprocessing

Disease, insect, and drug resistant crops
Healthier, more productive, disease resistant farm animals
More nutritious produce
Biopesticides
Edible vaccines incorporated into food products
New environmental cleanup uses for plants like tobacco

What do you know of the MMR vaccine?

Extract from http://hcd2.bupa.co..uk/fact_sheets/html/mmr.html

What is the MMR vaccine?
MMR is a combination vaccine that offers protection against three diseases:
Measles
Mumps
Rubella (German measles)
It is first given by injection, to children at around 13 months, with a second dose given as a preschool booster at around three to five years.1,2

The MMR vaccine can also be given to younger children, including babies from five months, who have been exposed to someone with a measles infection. This can prevent them from becoming ill themselves and helps to control the outbreak.
The first dose of the vaccine gives 90 percent protection against measles and mumps and 95 percent against rubella. This means that out of 100 people given the vaccine, 90 will then be immune to measles and mumps, and 95 to rubella. Adding a second dose increases the protection to over 99 percent for all three illnesses.1

Since the MMR vaccine was introduced in the UK in 1988, the

number of children catching measles, mumps and rubella has fallen to an all-time low. Until the recent scare no children have died from acute measles since 1992.

Autism and bowel disease
The speculation over a link between the MMR vaccine and autism started in 1998 when a paper was published in a medical journal about 12 autistic children who also had bowel problems. Although the research stated that they did not prove a link between autism and the MMR vaccine, the resulting publicity gave the impression that there was a link.

However, there is now a large body of scientific literature available, based on the records of millions of MMR vaccinations, that shows this is not the case. Based on this evidence, independent experts agree that there is no proven link between MMR and autism.

Although the number of cases of autism appears to have risen significantly in the last 20 years, this is probably due to better diagnosis of the condition, and a change in the way that doctors classify disorders so that autism is used more frequently than terms such as developmental delay.

What recent medical breakthroughs have arisen

There have been precious few medical break throughs in recent years. There is a great deal of research going on into stem cells and gene therapy but success has been elusive. Monoclonal antibody therapies help made a significant impact on diseases such as rheumatoid arthritis. Imaging has made significant strides and CT scans may reduce the need for therapies such as angiography (heart catheter insertion). Angiography and angioplasty, the passage of a catheter through an artery to the heart after which a balloon is inflated to unblock a coronary artery have largely replaced open heart surgery. Joint replacements have become more reliable and longer lasting. Most abdominal surgery is now done as keyhole day case surgery.

Statins to reduce cholesterol appear to be reducing heart disease albeit at considerable cost.

Which medical documentaries have you seen recently?
Obviously this will depend upon what has been shown recently. Expect to answer questions such as; what message was the producer trying to get across. Was it justified. Do you think this is a significant break through. What arguments might you put against the premise of the show?

What skills do you think are needed in order to communicate with your patients; how do you think they are best acquired?
How would you like your patients to describe you

These are really much the same question, positive behavioural indicators used in medical selection include;

Empathy/sensitivity; open, non judgemental, cooperative, warmth and encouragement, express ideas clearly, effective non verbal behaviour, humour, analogy.

You might then in your answer divide your answer into verbal and nonverbal communication skills. Nonverbal skills might include, listening, appropriate silence, nodding, nondefensive or aggressive body posture. Verbal skills include humour, analogy, clear description, negotiation, sensitivity and empathy.
Use these indicators in describing your skills

What interests do you bring from school/college life that you think will contribute to your studies and practice?
Have there been any particular life experiences that you think will help you in a career in medicine?

Obviously mention any sporting, artistic or musical expertise but think before hand how these might help you with medicine. You might have developed leadership skills as a captain or head of orchestra. You will have developed team working skills. You will have had to manage your time carefully and deal with multiple pressures. You will have developed communication and negotiation skills. If you have had to deal with adversity what inner strength or motivation did this result in? Artistic talent taught you patience and perseverance and a trained eye might be helpful in noticing clinical signs. I made you more dextrous and gave you an avenue to relief the stresses you might have developed.

What challenges do you think a career in medicine will bring you?
What do you think you will be the most negative aspects of being a doctor

Initially dealing with the volume of work that is required as a student and balancing work with life. Dealing with illness and death perhaps for the first time. Managing the demands of life as a junior doctor with long hours and considerable responsibility. Coping with the increase in litigation and the impact that has on ones self esteem. Dealing with uncertainty since medicine is an inexact science. The increasing expectations of the public and media and the access to often dubious medical information on the internet. The work can move quickly from the repetitive and mundane to highly stressful in a short period of time.

What do you think you will be the most positive aspects of being a doctor

Public respect is still high in spite of the Daily Mail! The subject is constantly changing and what ever career you follow in medicine you will need to continue your education in order to keep up. You will at times make a real difference and make a diagnosis that many would miss and by doing so save a life. You will work with a group of intelligent and stimulating people. Avoid commenting on salary!!

What attributes are necessary in a good doctor

The GMC defines a good doctor as;

Good doctors make the care of their patients their first concern: they are competent, keep their knowledge and skills up to date, establish and maintain good relationships with patients and colleagues, are honest and trustworthy, and act with integrity. There are opportunities to develop research and teaching skills and to manage departments or enter medical politics.

The duties of a doctor

The duties of a doctor registered with the General Medical Council Patients must be able to trust doctors with their lives and health. To justify that trust you must show respect for human life and you must:

Make the care of your patient your first concern
Protect and promote the health of patients and the public
Provide a good standard of practice and care
Keep your professional knowledge and skills up to date
Recognise and work within the limits of your competence
Work with colleagues in the ways that best serve patients' interests
Treat patients as individuals and respect their dignity
Treat patients politely and considerately
Respect patients' right to confidentiality
Work in partnership with patients
Listen to patients and respond to their concerns and preferences
Give patients the information they want or need in a way they can understand
Respect patients' right to reach decisions with you about their treatment and care

Support patients in caring for themselves to improve and maintain their health
Be honest and open and act with integrity
Act without delay if you have good reason to believe that you or a colleague may be putting patients at risk
Never discriminate unfairly against patients or colleagues
Never abuse your patients' trust in you or the public's trust in the profession.
You are personally accountable for your professional practice and must always be prepared to justify your decisions and actions.

<u>Which activities do you think you would like to do?</u>
<u>Would you like to do something new or continue your music/drama/mountaineering ?</u>
<u>What would you like people to remember about you from your medical school life?</u>
<u>The medical course is hard work. How do you propose to manage your work and still play football/violin ?</u>

Avoid saying that you recognise that you will have to work hard and so will give up your county level rugby. I have spoken to board members who 'phone their rugby captain or orchestra leader to ask what positions are required so do not reduce your chances by dropping a sport. You would like people to remember you as great fun, a real contributor to medical life, calm in adversity, someone who achieved their potential and the best second row the school has had for 10 years (insert sport or interest)

<u>Suggest how to reduce the costs of the NHS</u>
<u>If you were Alan Milburn what changes would you make to the NHS</u>

You might start to reduce health costs by using evidence based medicine to determine which treatments are successful and which may not be cost effective or effective. Look at switching people from branded drugs to generic drugs, branded drugs have a trade name and are more expensive, new drugs are branded until the patent runs out after which other companies can produce 'copycat' versions at reduced cost as they have not had to pay for the development of the drug.

Reduce the length of stay in hospital beds by improving community support or the number of nursing home beds.

Should we be made to pay for health care

Health care either has to be paid for by the state or by individuals. If the state funds the health care system as s the case in the NHS it is paid for by taxation. If the individual pays as is the case in the US, most people pay health insurance with the poorest being treated under a 'safety net system' called Medicare. Employers often pay insurance as a benefit so the burden falls on companies and so the economy. One can argue for both systems see page x

Do you know how different the health system is in e.g. France

The French health care system involves partial payment at the point of contact with a doctor, the state then refunds most if not all of the fee. General practitioners tend to work as groups of doctors all of whom have a special interest in one aspect of medicine such as child health or cardiology.

Comment on health care in developing countries

Health provision in the developing world is largely based in the towns and cities with poor rural provision, funding is poor and standards on he whole low. Much provision is via non governmental organisations that help with immunisation programmes.

If I gave you 10 million pounds for the NHS what would

you do

Ten million pounds does not go far in provision in health care. You have several options, you could fund a local project of your choice, perhaps health education in schools regarding diet, drugs, sexual health. You could contribute it the hospice movement in your area. You could buy some capital equipment, perhaps an MRI scanner, cardiac equipment. You could set up health provision for a developing country by attempting to provide clean water wells or immunisation for an area. National projects are out of your scope and you should point this out to indicate that you know of the cost in the NHS. The NHS budget runs into tens of <u>billions</u>.

What were the most recent NHS reforms

The most recent reforms in the NHS were MMC (see page x), choose and book page x), and payment by results.

Consultants contract why did they turn down a 24% increase
What do you think about doctor's private practice being reduced?

The consultants turned down the deal offered because it limited the amount of private work that they could perform for a relatively modest pay rise, some specialities that do little private work welcomed it.

Imagine you are on committee that has to recommend which of two new treatments can be made available through the NHS. On what grounds would you make your arguments?

You need to look at the cost of the two treatments in conjunction with the perceived benefit. If for instance one drug is expensive but is likely to cure 50% of those suffering from a previously untreatable common condition then the expense might be justified if previous treatments are made obsolete and there is a reduction in care costs in hospitals and hospices, outpatient blood testing and transfusions. You would also need to look at any risk associated with use of the two drugs. If it cured 20% of patients but killed 3% one would be seriously concerned about funding it. Does the drug require special training to administer, extra equipment or extra staff. How common are the diseases being targeted. Are there existing medications that are cheaper and just as effective? Have you looked at the evidence base for the treatment?

Which is more important general practice (primary care) or hospital, and why?

Take care not to leap in with hospitals as an answer. Consider the importance of general practice in preventative care and chronic disease monitoring. Consider also the efficiency of the primary care system in acting as a 'gatekeeper' to the secondary care sector. If patients were able to refer themselves to a consultant, think of the expense and wasted resources that might ensue. It is interesting that the US which has a private health care service has opted to adopt an NHS style 'family doctor' service, partly because patients value having one doctor as a first port of call but also because it saves the system money. On the other hand, if you have appendicitis or need a heart bypass you will not be able to have these performed in General Practice! There is though a move to shift non surgery (and some minor surgery) out of hospitals and into the community.

Do you think euthanasia should be legalised? Discuss the pros and cons. Should life be prolonged at all costs?

The views for and against are as follows;
For
Tremendous pain and suffering of patients can be saved.
The right to die should be a fundamental freedom of each person. Patients can die with dignity rather than have the illness reduce them to a shell of their former selves.

Health care costs can be reduced, which would save estates and lower insurance premiums.
Nurse and doctor time can be freed up to work on saveable patients.
Prevention of suicide is a violation of religious freedom.
Pain and anguish of the patient's family and friends can be lessened, and they can say their final goodbyes.
Reasonable laws can be constructed which prevent abuse and still protect the value of human life.
Vital organs can be saved, allowing doctors to save the lives of others.
Without physician assistance, people may commit suicide in a messy, horrifying, and traumatic way.

Against
 It would violate doctors' Hippocratic oath.
It demeans the value of human life.
It could open the floodgates to non critical patient suicides and other abuses.
Many religions prohibit suicide and the intentional killing of others.
Doctors and families may be prompted to give up on recovery much too early.
Insurance companies may put undue pressure on doctors to avoid heroic measures or recommend the assisted suicide procedure.
Miracle cures or recoveries can occur.
Doctors are given too much power, and can be wrong or unethical

Do you think the country needs more doctors or more nurses? What do you think will be the effects of having more female doctors than male doctors?

If you do think out your arguments carefully. The argument for more nurses is that trained nurses are so thin on the ground in hospital that they are put under undue pressure and this leads to sickness and people leaving the profession. Shift systems also make the job less attractive and again leads to loss of staff from the NHS which need to be replaced. However, bed numbers are falling due to shorter hospital stays and day case surgery. Nurses are also fulfilling many of the roles that doctors filled previously.

Nurse practitioners are working in hospital outpatients departments, G.P. surgeries and accident and emergency departments.

There is a steady shift toward a female medical work force, 6070% of doctors are now women. Many women wish to work part time and have families. This means that a retiring male doctor may need to be replaced by two female doctors. Some specialities are not conducive to a good work/life balance, particularly some of the surgical specialities like neurosurgery and transplant surgery. It may be very difficult to fill these roles in future years.

What are the arguments for and against banning the sale of tobacco?
Arguments for a ban. http://news.bbc.co..uk

Supporters of a ban say that evidence about the risks of passive smoking is too compelling to ignore. Some of the arguments they put forward are listed below.

Passive smoking is dangerous: Second hand smoking in the work place causes about 700 deaths each year, according to research from Imperial College.

A majority of people favour a smoking ban: A smoking ban in work places including pubs and bars is supported by a majority of people, according to a poll for the BBC in August 2004.

A ban would encourage more smokers to quit: A poll by Mintel in May 2004 found that 15 percent of smokers said they would quit smoking if a ban was introduced.

The "voluntary approach" has failed: The Wanless report on public health said the voluntary approach to smoking in the work place had only limited success pubs and bars still allow smoking.

People have a right to protect themselves from smoke inhalation: The British Medical Association argues that 70% of the population are currently denied the freedom to go about their lives in a smoke free environment.

Arguments against a ban
Opponents of a smoking ban say that freedom of choice would be affected. Some of the arguments they put forward are listed below:

People want restrictions not a ban: A Populous poll in May 2004 indicated that people would like to see restrictions on smoking rather than an outright ban.

People should have freedom of choice: The smokers' lobby group, Forest, points to a BBC poll which showed that 64% or people thought that smoking should be a personal matter.

Smoking bans damage business: A smoking ban could lead to a significant fall in takings from bars, restaurants and casinos. Licensed Victuallers Wales says the ban could lead to the closure of more than a quarter of pubs in Wales.

The link between passive smoking and ill health is unproven: Forest maintains there is no clear link between exposure to passive smoke and illness in nonsmokers. It has a briefing on the issue.

Self regulation is the solution: Left to market forces, pubs, bars and restaurants will introduce smoke free areas and better ventilation tailored to customers' needs, says Forest in a statement on the issue.

Why do doctors sometimes get a bad press?

There are a number of reasons. Some people resent what is seen as the power of doctors and perhaps, have an old fashioned view based on old films and the Daily Mail. Some doctors abuse their power and are seen as uncaring and dictatorial. Medicine is an emotive subject, if someone dies today, blame has to be attributed where once this was seen as part of the natural cycle of life.

There may be political reasons to try to diminish the support that doctors generally have amongst their patients. The medical lobby is powerful and the government have a vested interest in weakening it as it frequently speaks out against government policy. Changes in the out of hours care system are not universally popular although a recent questionnaire showed considerable satisfaction with patient access to a doctor

What is meant by the inequalities of health and what can be done to reduce them? http://www.dh.gov.uk/PolicyAnd-Guidance/fs/en

Inequalities exist on a number of levels. The North of the country has a lower average life span, higher neonatal mortality rates as do the poorest classes compared to the richest. Men have a lower life expectancy than do women. The government is attempting to reduce these gaps by reducing obesity, alcohol and smoking which are higher in the poor. Improving diet and encouraging exercise.

As a doctor, you have killed someone who otherwise would have survived how would you deal with that? What do you tell family

Do not forget to talk about your own feelings and how you would cope with this difficult situation. You will be upset and want to talk it through with colleagues and probably close family, maintaining confidentiality with regard to names. We all make mistakes but a doctor can make life threatening mistakes. There will be times when a diagnosis is only clear in retrospect and whereas the disease if picked up early might have been treatable it is the delay that was the problem. You will expect a local enquiry and possibly a coroner's inquest that is likely to be stressful. When dealing with the family, honesty is essential. Often complete honesty and a frank apology can be met with surprising understanding whereas a hint of a cover up will convince a family to pursue the case.

Jim is an alcoholic with end stage liver failure. His drinking is now under control but he needs a transplant. His local health authority refuses funding. What ethical issues does this raise?

This raises issues of autonomy in that the patient is being denied the right to choose their treatment option. Non-malifisense in that by not offering a transplant you are putting his life at risk. Justice in that the health authority have to make a decision on equitable distribution of funding. One is also going against GMC advice that we should not restrict access to treatment based on the fact that the condition is 'selfinflicted'?

A patient comes to you with a newspaper clipping suggesting that a new drug might be better than the one he takes. It is three times the cost to prescribe. What are the ethical issues raised.

Again speak of autonomy for the patient (a doctor can also have autonomy of course). Non-malifisense in that you might be denying a patient a better treatment. Justice, by prescribing the more expensive drug you are perhaps denying two other people the original drug.

Are you aware of any changes to the cervical screening program?

The cervical screening program is a program aimed at reducing deaths from cervical cancer and involves removing cells from the cervix or neck of the womb, looking at them under a microscope and assessing whether further treatment or investigation is needed. Recently the method has changed to a liquid based cytology that is more accurate and produces less false negative and repeat tests but is more expensive.

What are your views on genetic testing and insurance?

There are two issues here, the first is the availability of genetic tests undertaken for health reasons to insurance companies. The second is the possibility that in the future insurance companies will ask people to undergo testing prior to accepting them. An example might be Huntingdon's Disease a fatal degenerative disease that affects 50% of children of families carrying the gene. The reason there is an ethical issue here is that patients underwent the testing, perhaps to assess breast cancer risk, in good faith and without expecting it to fall into the hands of insurers who will assess risk and possibly decline their insurance request. This has serious implications if one cannot insure ones life to protect your family.

Everyone knows that doctors treat ill people. What else do you think doctors do?

Doctor perform occupational health work which involves health and safety advice to businesses. They work for medical defence unions and insurance companies offering advice on risk and claims. They provide services to patients in order to prevent disease for example secondary prevention of heart disease in a diabetic. They can be medical politicians working for the British Medical Association or advising the government. They can help in the administration of hospitals or as educationalists or researchers.

What health problems are encountered in East London.

This might be asked by one of the London Hospitals but others may mention an area of deprivation near their own hospital. It is aimed to test your knowledge of the area and of epidemiology. Deprived areas have increased levels of smoking related disease, coronary heart disease, lung cancer, bladder cancer and chronic obstructive pulmonary disease (bronchitis and emphysema as it was once known). Obesity is greater and with it the risk of diabetes. Diseases related to poor nutrition and immigration such as tuberculosis.

Lower employment rates lead to higher depression rates. Life expectancy is reduced.

Is the NHS in crisis?

This is a reference to the constant media message that the NHS is going to the dogs. It is not, in reality the patient experience has improved enormously with shorter waiting lists, more doctors, massive investment. The new deal for consultants and General practitioners was miscalculated by the government who underestimated the cost and then said that they had pumped enough into the NHS and it would have to find the increased expenditure out of existing funds. This led to wholesale cuts in staff, mainly nurses and administrators but doctors also. Changes to working practices have meant that because doctors are only allowed to work a set number of hours (see EWTD), more doctors are needed to cover 24 hour care. NHS inflation is much higher than general inflation as new developments lead to expensive new capital equipment costs. Changes related to MMC mean that there are fewer specialist posts available for training but in reality many people who eventually enter general practice start in a speciality and so MMC merely formalises training so that people make a career decision at an earlier stage, which some may see as a disadvantage. What has changed is that the power wielded by consultants has diminished in favour of managers who doctors often perceive as being bean counters disinterested in the care of patients and more interested in balancing the books. This naturally leads to conflict.

When was the NHS formed, who was the first minister for the NHS
http://www.nhs.uk/england/aboutTheNHS/history/default.cmsx

The National Health Service became reality on 5 July 1948. Aneurin Bevan was the first minister. Food was still rationed, building materials were short, there was a dollar economic crisis and a shortage of fuel. The war had created a housing crisis alongside postwar rebuilding of cities, and the designation of overspill areas, the New Towns Act (1946) created major new centres of population and all needed health services.

Administrative difficulties

The NHS brought hospital services, family practitioner services (doctors, pharmacists, opticians and dentists) and community based services into one organisation for the first time. But it was not easy. Holding everything together and keeping everyone on board continued to create administrative difficulties for years.

Costs

Financial problems, however, were worse. It was impossible to predict the day-to-day costs of the new service and public expectations rose. Medical science was rapidly gathering pace, hospital beds for tuberculosis were closed, allowing cash to be released for other services.

More mothers were wanting their babies delivered in hospital, cardiac surgery was being applied to rheumatic heart disease, and the first hip replacements were beginning to be performed.

But initial estimates of the cost of the NHS were soon exceeded as newer, more expensive and more frequently used drugs were developed.

Fees

Within three years of its creation, the NHS, which had been conceived as free of direct charges for everyone, was forced to introduce some modest fees. Prescription charges of one shilling (5p), which had been legislated for as early as 1949 but had not been implemented, were introduced in 1952. A flat rate of £1 for ordinary dental treatment was brought in at the same time.

Balancing demands

Many of the tensions that emerged in the early days of the NHS have challenged its senior management and successive Governments ever since. Today the NHS has a work force of over one million people and a budget of around £42 billion year it is a sophisticated and modern organisation with all the advantages of state-of-the-art technology. Yet, the fundamental questions that tested Bevan and his colleagues how best to organise and manage the service, how to fund it adequately, how to balance the often conflicting demands and expectations of patients, staff and taxpayers, how to ensure finite resources are targeted where they are most needed continue to challenge the system.

Bevan foresaw this. We shall never have all we need he said. Expectations will always exceed capacity. The service must always be changing, growing and improving it must always appear inadequate.

Family doctors

The foundation of the new service was the family doctor or general practitioner (G.P.). Then, as now, the family doctor acted as gatekeeper to the rest of the NHS, referring patients where appropriate to hospitals or specialist treatment and prescribing medicines and drugs.

Dental services consisted of checkups and all necessary fillings and dentures. There was a school dental service and a special priority service for expectant and nursing mothers and young children that was organised by local authorities. Eye tests were provided by ophthalmic opticians on production of a G.P. referral note.

Community health

A major innovation was the community health centres a special premise with accommodation and equipment supplied from public funds to enable family doctors, dentists and others to work together to provide a range of services on the spot. There were also specialist ear clinics at which patients could get an expert opinion and, if needed, a new hearing aid.

Why do we need screening and how do we carry it out.

Screening tests should be cheap, screen for important diseases, have few false positives and few false negatives and should screen for a disease you can treat otherwise it is rather pointless. We currently have national screening programmes for breast cancer with mammograms, cervical cancer with smear tests , babies are screened with blood tests a week after birth to detect hypothyroidism (cretinism) and a rare genetic defect, The other organised screening test is of pregnant women, at about 11 weeks gestation, nuchal fold ultrasound scans are performed on the mothers to look at the neck of the baby where measurements are taken and combined with a blood test to estimate the risk of a Downs syndrome baby, .There are screening tests for bowel cancer with colonoscopy and prostate cancer with the PSA blood test but these are not organised programmes and target symptomatic cases on the whole.

Are there exams after university, what are they? Describe the path after medical school

The exams after medical school depend upon your speciality. You will have organised appraisal with each job and will have to show competence in each given field. As mentioned earlier you will have six four month foundation posts in different specialities. You will then move to specialist training schemes. In medicine you will take the MRCP, Membership of the Royal College of Physicians, for surgery the FRCS, Fellowship of the Royal College of Surgeons, for General Practice, Membership of the Royal College of G.P.s other specialities have their own membership examinations. You will then move to higher specialist training or move into General Practice, before taking up Consultant posts (which may be Junior or Senior)

Senior Medical Appointments

Specialist and GP training programmes (3-6 years)

F2 year

F1 year

Medical School 4-5 years

Simplified version of Modernising Medical Careers

What do you think of nurses developing extended roles and undertaking tasks previously done by doctors? What do you think about the proposal that nurses could replace doctors as the first contact person in primary care?

Specialist nurses are taking an increasing role in Hospitals and General Practice, they undertake specialist training to take on the role of diabetes liaison nurses to train people to give them selves insulin and adjust their dosing, rheumatology to inject joints and monitor disease, dermatology to perform minor operations and accident and emergency to act as triage nurses and nurse practitioners, applying plaster casts and managing many of the medical problems in minor injuries units. In General Practice they undertake an additional three year training to manage many of the cases presenting in surgeries and can prescribe a limited range of drugs. They are cheaper to employ than doctors but have a more limited training. Some studies suggest though that they take longer to deal with problems and so may not always be a cheaper option.

Tell us what attracts you most and least about this Medical School

This can be a tricky one, the reason you chose it could also be a disadvantage. If it is traditional rather than a PBL school you could mention the delay in patient contact or the limitations of PBL but follow it up with ' I recognised this when I applied but on balance feel it is the type of learning that best suits me'.
You might say that the placements can be a long way from the university but that this is balanced by the variety of placements offered. It could be near to home (this can be a disadvantage), cost can be an issue. See the section on choosing a medical school for other pros and cons.

"You are the head of panel for the proposition of changing every London taxi to vehicles with Hybrid engines. What

would you include in your report?".

This was a slightly wacky question from Keele who have a reputation for scientific questions. You will probably start with a medical viewpoint. Reducing emissions will reduce the amount of CO_2, diesel particles that are thought to cause respiratory problems such as worsening asthma and chronic airways disease. Scientists believe highly reactive metals and chemical groups in the diesel soot particles interfere with the normal function of blood vessels, reducing their ability to relax effectively, a process that eventually leads to them hardening and thickening.
The electrical energy would require generators but these can be clean burning and less polluting. You could mention other green energies such as hydrogen and plant derived fuels. You would have to balance this with the economic cost of changing engines that would be passed on to the customer and lead to other modes of transport being used. This could be beneficial if greener but it could result in personal cars being used.
Hybrid cars use braking energy to recharge batteries and the engines switch off when not moving thus saving more fuel.

What is The path after Medical school and what are the arguments for and against MMC?

The Foundation Programme is a two year general training programme that forms the bridge between medical school and specialist/general practice training. Trainees will have the opportunity to gain experience in a series of placements in a variety of specialities and health care settings. Learning objectives for each stage will be specific and focused on demonstration of clinical competencies.

Foundation Year 1 (F1)

The first year of the Foundation Programme builds upon the knowledge, skills and competencies acquired in undergraduate training. The learning objectives for this year are set by the General

Medical Council. In order to attain full registration with the GMC, doctors must achieve specific competencies by the end of this year. (See the GMC website for more details: www.gmcuk.org)

Foundation Year 2 (F2)

Typically, F2 placements will be allocated during the first year to afford doctors in training and their supervisors some flexibility and choice in response to early training experiences.

The second year of the Foundation Programme builds on the first year of training. The F2 year main focus is on training in the assessment and management of the acutely ill patient. Training also encompasses the generic professional skills applicable to all areas of medicine team work, time management, communication and IT skills.

The BMA (British Medical Association) the doctors trade union have a number of concerns about MMC;

Their website lists them as follows;
1, The delay in submission of curricula by several Royal Colleges has raised concerns that the information necessary for selection will not be adequate.

2, There is deep concern for the lack of flexibility within the current MMC plans.

3, The MTAS frontend user interface appears to be easy to use, and, as described to JDC, the hardware backing it up should be robust enough to cope with the peak demand as people apply. However, the underlying application process still has a worryingly short timetable as well as very short periods of notice for attending interviews and accepting or rejecting offers made.

4, A further reason to support delay is to allow enough time for additional selection tools to be developed, piloted, validated, and for training in their use to be disseminated.

5, With fierce competition for places, applicants will need to attend all their interviews within a short period. Simultaneous disruptions to service and clashing interviews do not, as yet, appear to have been taken into consideration. .

6, Doctors at this stage in their training are required to make a momentous decision regarding not only their training but their future career. It is feared that the proposed level of careers guidance and counselling will not be sufficient or timely for this year's recruitment.

7, The indicative number of RTG (run through grade) posts and fixedTerm Specialist Training Appointments (FTSTAs) for the UK has been announced in early October as 22,000 to 23,000, with 17,000 to 18,000 offering "access to run through training". Firmer figures have been promised in December 2006. This is a substantial improvement on the 9,500 posts for England confirmed earlier, but still leaves a shortfall.

8, Inadequate work force planning has lead to uninformed decisions with regards to the number of NTNs available within each speciality. This information must be accurate.

The arguments made for MMC are;

Modernising Medical Careers (MMC) aims to improve patient care by delivering a modernised and focused career structure for doctors through a major reform of postgraduate medical education. It aims to develop demonstrably competent doctors who are skilled at communicating and working as effective members of a team. As training and education are central to the work of doctors and their role in delivering patient care, MMC will also bring about significant changes to career structures, providing qualified staff who are able to meet the needs of patients.

The two year foundation schools will, for the first time, require doctors to demonstrate their abilities and competence against set standards. There will be an opportunity to develop experience in a range of specialities. This will offer doctors the chance to gain insight into possible career options or to build a wider appreciation of medicine before embarking on specialist training.

Postfoundation, specialist/G.P. training will be streamlined to deliver specialists who are judgement safe and able to deliver the care that is needed to treat patients, without compromising in any way on standards. Streamlined training will also afford further opportunities for super specialisation that are flexible enough to allow doctors to adapt to accommodate changes in medical technology. In this way the new system under MMC aims to provide the right numbers of doctors to meet changing service needs.

Streamlined training and explicit standards of assessed competence are also essential if doctors' careers are to accommodate the pressures of a family and modern lifestyles. MMC aims to greatly improve the opportunities for those who wish to take a break in their careers and will promote fairness and equality of opportunity at all stages of a doctors' career.

Modernising Medical Careers is also a key enabler for other flagship programmes in the Department of Health. It is focused on the development of a flexible work force of doctors, who are both competent at dealing with the acutely ill and who are effective at communicating with patients and colleagues alike. These skills and the absolute guarantee of standards from new methods of assessment are key to the success of modern work force programmes like the Hospital at Night, and the Working Time Directive. Most importantly, however, MMC will deliver a modern training scheme and career structure that will allow clinical professionals to support real patient choice.

The above is taken from the MMC website. Reading between the lines the message is 'we were told to train more doctors quickly. In order to do this we have shortened the training but to protect ourselves from the charge of under training doctors we will record competencies as they go along so that we can prove it is not our fault!' The biggest complaint is from surgeons who claim it is not possible to train a surgeon adequately in the time allotted given the limits to working hours ruled by the EWTD.

What is confidentiality? When can a doctor breach confidentiality?

Rules of confidentiality (studentBMJ 2006;14:353-396 October)

Patients have a right to expect that their doctors will keep information about them in strict confidence. As part of the privilege of the doctor-patient relationship, the doctor has a responsibility to protect the patient's right to confidentiality. This has led to a series of rules that doctors must be aware of and follow in their clinical practice. But, as for all rules, circumstances exist when they may be broken for good reason, and doctors must also be aware of these exceptions.

Rights and responsibilities
Being registered as a medical practitioner gives doctors rights and privileges. In return, doctors have a duty to meet standards of competence, care, and conduct. This includes maintaining patients' confidentiality, which is central to the trust between doctors and patients. Without the assurance of confidentiality, patients may be reluctant to provide comprehensive information required for optimal health care.
It is often taken for granted that patients give "implied consent" to medical information being disclosed to others for "health care purposes." Fortunately, most patients understand that information

must be shared within the health care team that is providing the treatment.

Rules of disclosure

Inform patients about the disclosure, or check that they have already received information about it
Anonymise data if unidentifiable data will serve the purpose
Be satisfied that patients know about disclosures necessary to provide their care so that they can object to these disclosures if they wish
Seek patients' express consent to disclosure information, where identifiable data are needed for any purpose other than the provision of care or for clinical audit
Keep disclosures to the minimum necessary
Keep up to date with and observe the requirements of statute and common law, including data protection legislation. These requirements may differ between countries and are likely to change over time.
Pitfalls...

Most breaches of confidentiality occur "inadvertently" in settings such as ward rounds in cubicles with multiple beds and overheard "discussions management" in corridors.
You should not leave patients' records, either on paper or on screen, where they can be seen by other patients, unauthorised health care staff, or the public. The area of electronic health records has increased the opportunity for breaching a patient's right to confidentiality.1

You must still keep information confidential after a patient dies. Requests for information after a patient's death may be complex and cause distress or benefit to the patient's family. The purpose of the disclosure should be clear, and you should seek legal advice.

Reasons to disclose information
These criteria may vary between countries make sure you know the rules in your country

Health care reasons

Parents (when child is unable to give informed consent)
Care givers or family of patients with intellectual impairment or dementia

Public interest
Where there is risk of serious harm or death to the patient or other people
Provisions in the Mental Health Act
Required by law

Court ordered by the health ombudsman or coroner
Complaints committees
Child abuse
Serious criminality
Medically unfit patients continuing to drive despite advice
Required by statutory regulatory bodies

Notifiable diseases
Drug addiction
Termination of pregnancy
Births and deaths
Identification of patients undergoing in vitro fertility treatment with donated gametes (and the outcome of such treatment)
Identification of donors and recipients of transplanted organs
Prevention, apprehension, or prosecution of terrorists
.. and exceptions

Various situations may arise in which you might be legally and ethically obliged to breach confidentiality and disclose information about a patient in your care. These primarily relate to disclosure in connection with judicial or other statutory proceedings, disclosure in the public interest to protect either the patient or others, or in circumstances when children or other patients may lack competence to give consent.

If you consider that a legal or ethical requirement to divulge information exists, as a junior doctor you should discuss this with a senior clinician in conjunction with the hospital's legal advisers. When this is done, the patient should be informed wherever possible, but not if there are concerns of violence or danger to other people. Disclosures should be kept to the minimum amount of information necessary for the purpose.

Learning through examples

HIV from an affair. Your patient has requested an HIV test after a high risk extramarital affair. The test result comes back positive. He urges you to keep the test result a secret, in particular from his wife who he is convinced will leave him if she finds out about the affair. He refuses to use barrier contraception as his wife would become suspicious.

The patient should be urged to tell his wife and given the opportunity to control the release of this information. However, you have a responsibility to tell the wife because her life is being placed in danger by his actions. In this case, his conduct poses a risk to others that outweighs his right to medical confidentiality. After repeated counselling, discussion with senior colleagues, and both the Medical Protection Society and the General Medical Council, you advise his wife accordingly and inform the patient that you have done so.

Driver with epilepsy A patient has recently been diagnosed as having epilepsy. You inform him of his obligation to notify the road transport authority, which will probably revoke his licence. He tells you that he has no intention of doing this because he will lose his job as a travelling salesman.

The road transport authority must be notified because the salesman is putting other drivers at risk. The road transport authority has the responsibility of deciding if someone is medically unfit to drive. The authority needs to know when drivers have a condition that might affect their safety or the safety of other people. If a patient has a condition which may affect their ability to drive, you should explain this to them and ask them to inform the road transport authority. If they refuse to do so, you must inform the road transport authority and let the patient know that you have done so.

Release of information   A patient in your care is being investigated for a malignancy. The patient's best friend approaches you in visiting hours and asks you how he is getting on and what the tests have shown.

You should absolutely not divulge information about the patient's medical condition to the friend without the express consent of the patient. If the patient does consent, any discussion with the friend should take place with the patient present. This would apply equally to a family member.

Taking medical records home   You are required to present a case at the weekly departmental meeting and do not have enough time to prepare your presentation while at work. So you take the hospital case notes home over the weekend, but unfortunately the medical records were in your briefcase, which is stolen from your car.

Bad mistake and bad luck. To ensure that patient information is protected, records must be kept physically secure at all times. As a result, hospitals normally have a standard rule that staff cannot take patient records home. In addition to the risk of loss, such an action may also adversely affect patients' care should they be readmitted and the records are not available.

Disclosure to employers and insurance companies.   You receive a request from a patient's employer to confirm the dates and details of hospital admission six weeks after the patient has been discharged. The patient had been admitted with pneumonia and there were no "sensitive issues."

You need to get consent from the patient to release this personal information, even though there seems to be no sensitive issue. The same principle applies to requests for information from insurance companies.

Patients younger than 16 years old. A 14 year old girl attends the emergency department to get a prescription for the oral contraceptive pill. She does not want to see her normal general practitioner that she fears will tell her parents. She asks you not to inform her parents. What should you do?

If you consider that the patient is competent to consent to treatment and requests that the treatment is prescribed without the knowledge of her parents, her wishes should be respected. And it is legal to do so. But you should ensure that you provide the patient with sexual health advice and encourage her to accept long term follow up with a general practitioner.

Serious crime A patient attends the emergency department with a gunshot injury that requires surgery. He says that it was an unintentional injury he got when cleaning his shotgun. You are aware of a media report of an armed hold up in a neighbouring town, in which one of the assailants was shot by his mate and in which a shop assistant was beaten up.

You are obliged to tell the police because this represents a "serious crime," in which another person suffered "serious harm." It is best to discuss the case with a consultant, who would need to take responsibility for contacting the police.

How would you cope with a difficult patient? What types are there?

The "difficult patient" (studentBMJ 2006;14:265-308 July)

Every doctor encounters patients who are frustrating and dissatisfying to look after. It has been estimated that these patients make up as much as 15% of our clinical practice. Junior doctors should recognise that although the "difficult patient" has multiple guises, the syndrome does exist, it is not uncommon, and certain management strategies and support are available to help.

It is also worth recognising that patients may sometimes encounter a "difficult doctor." This is likely to occur if the doctor has the unfortunate characteristics of narcissism, arrogance, and poor communication skills.

How do we recognise the difficult patient?

Understanding the difficult patient has come a long way since 1978, when Groves described them as "hateful patients" and proposed four distinct stereotypes: the dependent clinger, the entitled demander, the manipulative help rejecter, and the self destructive denier.

It is now recognised that they are a disparate group of patients with a wide range of characteristics and behaviours, of which only a few may be present in any one patient. Often, there is a degree of personality disorder or abnormal behaviour engendered by chronic physical illness. Seemingly the personality disorder may have gone unrecognised.

How does it affect the doctor

Difficult patients have a common characteristic of causing doctors distress over a considerable period of time. Some patients behave in a way for which doctors are totally unprepared such as verbal abuse, harassment, and unfounded complaints. If doctors respond to a patient in a manner outlined in box 2, they are likely to be attending a difficult patient requiring particular care.

Box 1: Characteristics of the difficult patient

Multiple (unexplained) physical symptoms
Frequent attending
Somatisation disorder
Breaks doctor-patient boundaries
Won't or can't get better sick role issues
Noncompliance (including treatment)
Believes doctors are gods
Hostility and signing out
Litigious
Manipulative
Has (undiagnosed) personality disorder (borderline or dependent)
May have chronic medical disorders or social disabilities
Chronic pain syndromes with or without drug addiction
What is the source of the problem?

When dealing with a difficult patient the first thing to do is to identify the source of the problem. Is it primarily due to the patient, the doctor, or the patient-doctor relationship, or is it due to the health care system?

Failures within the doctor-patient relationship include poor communication with the patient and not recognising what the patient wants. Difficulties may emanate from the junior doctor not recognising how the patient copes with his or her disease or not understanding what the disease means for the patient.

Problems within the health care system outside the control of the junior doctor may contribute. On the wards there may be a lack of attention or adequate time to spend with the patient because of excessive workload. In the outpatient department the doctor may be "on the back foot" from the start because of the clinic running late or previous appointments having been cancelled. Lack of continuity of care may be a problem in both the inpatient and outpatient setting as a result of shift work and multiple responsibilities.

Box 2: Doctors' responses to difficult patients

Avoidance
Frustration
Anger
Anxiety
Prejudice
Defeat
What approaches can be taken?

Box 3: Management strategies for difficult patients

Consolidate the clinical team (for example, discuss at multi disciplinary team meetings)
Attend the patient as a team where possible (avoid splitting)
Set limits
Have a clear management plan and communicate it
Consider psychiatric input (early)
Acknowledge social issues as well as medical issues
Maintain professional standards despite manipulation
Give clear feedback on test results
Educate yourself on cultural aspects of illness
Maintain respect (despite the difficulties)
Avoid a judgmental approach (which may be difficult)
Be honest (including diagnostic or treatment issues and unmet expectations)
Consider treatment "contract" (health care agreement)

What one question would you ask if interviewing others interested in studying medicine?

Pick one that you wish to answer as the supplementary is likely to be 'how would you answer that?'. You might choose 'what do you think you can offer the school' knowing you can launch into a eulogy of your abilities. Or choose something you have prepared such as 'what qualities do you think a doctor should have'.

What are the health implications of global warming? see page 70

What are the arguments for and against cloning

Twenty-one Arguments Against Human Cloning, And Their Responses (http://www.genesage.com/professionals/geneletter/archives/twentyonearguments.html). You may disagree with these sentiments but they will provoke thought and give you an idea of the arguments that may be posed at interview.

1. argument: cloning is an affront to human dignity.

response: usually people who make this argument are unable to explain why cloning offends human dignity. the argument is supposed to be self-evident. the argument is based on "genetic essentialism", or "genetic determinism" a belief that one's unique humanness is entirely a product of one's dna. the argument is reductionist and itself an affront to human dignity. it is somewhat ironic that the unesco declaration on the human genome, after stating clearly that people should not be equated with their genes, goes on to say, without explanation, that cloning is an affront to human dignity.

2. argument: cloning is unnatural.

response: nature creates clones all the time, as identical twins. this happens in about 3 1/2 to 4 births per 1,000. twins ordinarily think of themselves as individuals, not as carbon copies of someone else. identical twins differ in many respects. they have different life expectancies, fingerprints, iq's (by up to 20 points), risks for schizophrenia (if one has schizophrenia, there is a 30% chance that the other will not), sexual orientations (concordance for homosexuality ranges from 0% to 100%, depending on the research study) and chances of criminal behaviour (concordance is about 50%, almost the same as for fraternal or dizygotic twins, indicating that environment may be the determining factor).

identical twins differ for the following reasons:

1. an embryo may divide at any time up to about 14 days after conception.
2. x-chromosome inactivation (lionisation) in early female embryos randomly turns off one x-chromosome in each cell. when an embryo "twins", the halves may contain different proportions of paternal and maternal x-chromosomes.
3. "genetic imprinting" (the process that marks which genes are be activated) in early embryos is variable.
even conjoined twins are different from each other. eng and chang bunker, the original "siamese twins", had different personalities. one was a depressed alcoholic, the other a cheerful teetotaler. they married separate wives, alternated living in separate houses, and fathered 21 children. abigail and brittany hensel share a common body below the neck, but feel sleepy or hungry at different times and may get different grades in school.
clones would not be as alike as twins, because clones would have different developmental signals from the different eggs from which they develop, different mitochondria from the eggs, different prenatal environments (e.g., maternal nutrition, toxic exposure), and different postnatal environments, including family and historical period.

3. argument: it's all right if nature makes clones, but if we do it we're "playing god".
response: modern medicine rarely leaves matters to "nature". we use ivf, try to keep 700-gram newborns alive, and, where culture and religion permit, use donor sperm, eggs, or embryos. why is cloning different from other reproductive technologies?

4. argument: clones will not have individual souls.
response: theologians of all religions agree that clones will each have

individual souls.

5. argument: clones will be treated as second-rate, because they're "carbon copies". isn't this an affront to dignity?
response: this is a "science fiction" view. do twins feel "second rate" because each looks like the other?

6. argument: clones will become increasingly inferior, as more copies of the same individual are produced.
response: this is the "photocopy machine" argument. there's no scientific evidence for it. it's unlikely that clones will be mass-produced. women have to bear them and someone has to raise them. this is an important point that much discussion about cloning overlooks.

7. argument: cloning uses a human being as a means to an end.
response: parents have children for many reasons, both selfish and unselfish. the same would be true of cloning, but why should it be subject to special rules? if society examines people's motives for parenthood and gives them "licenses" to become parents, this would give governments dictatorial powers.
sometimes it may be ethically allowable to conceive a child primarily for the benefit of someone else, as long as the child is loved and cared for as an equal with a family's other children. this has already occurred, when parents of a teenager with leukemia conceived a child as a marrow donor. consider the following case, which actually happened in the united states. case: conceiving a child to benefit a teenager with leukaemia.

a couple have a teenager with leukaemia. she will die within 2 to 3 years without a bone marrow transplant. the parents cannot find a donor with compatible marrow, so they conceive a baby in the hope that the baby will have marrow suitable for a transplant. there is a one-in-four chance that the baby's marrow will be compatible.

when asked on a survey, without knowing the case's outcome, 65% of u.s. genetics patients (n=476) and 52% of the u.s. public (n=988) approved the couple's decision. in the actual case, the baby had compatible marrow, the teenager's life was saved and the parents were happy with their new baby.

8. argument: cloning will be used to create armies or slaves.
response: armies and slaves can be created faster and more cheaply by other means than cloning. women are necessary to bear and raise the clones, and most will not be willing.

9. argument: wealthy people will clone themselves to have organ banks of "spare parts" in case they need hearts or livers. these clones could be made without heads, so they could be killed for organs without committing murder.

response: using another person for "spare parts" is murder and would be prosecuted as such. clones are undeniably persons. making "headless clones" to supply organs would also be murder. it would require decerebrating (removing the higher brain) of a fetus or infant. since the fetus or infant falls under the same legal/ethical rules as a non-cloned fetus or infant, whoever did this would be prosecuted. furthermore, there is no need to create an entire human. individual tissues or organs could be grown.

10. argument: parents (or societies) will have unrealistic expectations of clones. a clone of beethoven would be expected to produce an equivalent of the ninth symphony. a father might expect his clone to be his equal in sports. everyone will suffer if clones do not live up to expectations.

response: parents may have unrealistic expectations in the absence of cloning. cloning may reduce these expectations. a cloned parent who is clumsy will not expect the child to excel in sports.

11. argument: cloning will create new forms of the family.

response: true, but are these necessarily harmful? just because a family relationship is new and untried is not a reason to condemn it automatically. in the past, well-meaning policymakers have condemned as harmful many types of family relationships later shown to cause no harm to the children. in the united states, family constellations that most lawyers and ethicists considered harmful 20 years ago are now accepted. these include:

joint custody of children after divorce
single motherhood
single fatherhood
single-parent adoption
interracial adoption
lesbian and gay parenting

none of these has been shown to harm children, provided that enough economic resources are available. (poor families, whatever their structure, usually do not do as well).

12. argument: existence of "twins" (or triplets, etc.) a generation apart may be psychologically harmful to all.

response: this is one of the best arguments against cloning. we cannot predict psychosocial outcomes accurately. we have no idea what it would be like to grow up as the child of a parent who seems to know you "from inside", having gone through many of your own emotional crises in the same way. to the extent that sentiment, sadness, happiness, shyness, and other psychological characteristics may be biologically based, the parent will know in advance what crises a cloned teenager will go through and how he or she will respond. we need to ask ourselves whether we really want this degree of intimacy, which may border on extrasensory perception. It may produce a good and loving relationship, because the parent may understand, to greater degree than most parents, what the child is going through. On the other hand, most children want to have their own "secret places" where the parent cannot fathom what they think. The parent may impose expectations on the child, failing to realize that things may turn out very differently in a new historical period.

In some cases, people may decide to clone one of their own parents or grandparents instead of themselves. The psychosocial implications of raising a clone of one's parent are particularly unsettling. However, people may adjust more easily to new kinship arrangements than we think.

There is no reason to prejudge potential families with cloned children. As with adoption, in-vitro fertilization, and use of donor sperm, how the child will react to the news about his/her mode of arrival in the world will depend to a large extent on how the parents themselves feel about this mode of reproduction. If they are at ease with it, the child will be too. If they are not, there may be problems. Parents and children may adjust to cloning far more easily than we think, just as has happened with in-vitro fertilization. Predictions about dire psychosocial harms from ivf and other new reproductive technologies have turned out to be wrong.

13. Argument: people will abandon sexual reproduction in favor of cloning.
This is ridiculous, in view of financial costs. Also, cloning is no fun. Most couples prefer a child related to both, not one.

14. Argument: people may be cloned surreptitiously, against their will.
Response: true. Blood taken for medical purposes or hair left at the barbershop could be stolen. Laws may be necessary to prevent this by requiring the consent of any person who is cloned (or of the parents, if the individual is a child). In the united states, civil lawsuits (for monetary damages) might be a deterrent.

15. Argument: cloning "commodifies" children.
Response: all reproductive technologies, and adoption, cost money. This does not make a baby less valuable to its parents or reduce the amount of love they give it. Below is a price list of what various reproductive alternatives cost.

Ivf $10,000-12,000
Donor egg $5,000
Adoption of healthy white infant $25,000-40,000
Surrogate mother $45,000
Cloning? $100,000 ?

16. Argument: cloning will increase social inequalities, because only the richest will be able to afford it.
Response: an excellent argument. But this is true of all new reproductive technologies (nrts) and also of prenatal diagnosis. Differential use of nrts could increase existing differences between classes in health and longevity. The only way to prevent this is a universal health care system guaranteeing equal access to even the most expensive nrts and restricting their use to infertility that cannot be treated otherwise.

17. Argument: cloning is unsuccessful. "Only 1 in 277 tries" succeeded for wilmut.
Response: wilmut's actual statistics: 277 nuclear fusions led to 29 embryos, implanted in 13 ewes, of which 1 gave birth. One in 13 is a higher "success rate" than ivf had during its development and early years.

18. Argument: cloning is unsafe.
Cloning will produce damaged children, because the cells of an adult human have been exposed to environmental toxins for many years and have developed new mutations. Children may age and die rapidly because the chromosomes in an adult have shortened telomeres (end points of a chromosome that shorten with each cell division, until the cell is no longer able to divide), a result of cellular aging.

Response: animal experiments are necessary to answer these questions. It would be unethical to proceed with human cloning until animal experiments have proved its safety.

19. Argument: cloning is a denial of death.

Response: so is having children in the usual way, at least in some cultures. In the old testament, which had no belief in an afterlife, one of the greatest blessings god could bestow was that one's descendants would live long upon the earth. In china, one has a duty to have children in order to "keep one's ancestors alive". The clone does not carry one's consciousness or soul into the future, only one's genes. Therefore it is hard to see how this is a greater denial of death than simply having children.

20. Argument: cloning "feels wrong". It produces powerful negative emotions.
Response feelings alone are not an adequate foundation for ethics. Many people "feel it's wrong" for members of different races to marry or even live near each other. Historically, "feelings" about inherent rights and wrongs have been used to justify racial and social segregation and oppression, among other evils. Feelings have a place in ethics, but need to be examined by careful reasoning.

21. Argument: cloning could reduce human diversity, especially if carried out on a large scale.
Response: this is unlikely with humans, though it could occur with domestic animals. Most people want to have children who are the biological offspring of both or at least one parent, not the clone of some famous individual. Mass cloning of famous or wealthy individuals who want to populate the earth could be prevented by regulations that would stipulate that the number of cloned children could not exceed the maximum that would ordinarily survive in nature, probably five (quintuplets) or the number now allowed by most sperm banks (ten). It appears extremely doubtful that anyone would attempt such mass cloning, except in a totalitarian society. Families would have to accept and rear the cloned embryos, and the experience of sperm banks suggests that most people do not want the children of famous people, but want healthy children who are like themselves.

How do you think the rise in information technology has influenced and will influence the practice of medicine?

There are a number of in initiatives here. Past developments are access to the internet has offered educational opportunities such as access to journals, medical search engines, ebooks, medical websites. IT in general practice has allowed accurate recording of information and searching of notes in order to develop disease databases which are now used for quality monitoring. In hospitals, xrays are now viewed on computer screens rather than films and so can be viewed at home or another site.

'Choose and book' is mentioned elsewhere and is a means of GPs booking appointments at hospital and offering choice of several hospitals to a patient. Improved IT recording has made 'payment by results' a possibility by improved access to records of work performed. IT has allowed the development of special scans such as CT and MRI scans. Angiography and angioplasty require the use of sophisticated software and xray equipment. Software protocols are used to assist with chronic disease management and the data recorded automatically inserted into the records.

The future will see more telemedicine where consultations are performed with the doctor and patient or doctor and doctor in different sites. There is already the technology available to perform surgery via a robot some way away from the surgeon.

Ten years ago most doctors in hospitals wore white coats; now few do. Why do you think this is? What do you think are the arguments for and against white coats?

Arguments for;
they offer protection against bodily fluids
if changed regularly they prevent home clothes being contaminated
they are a uniform allowing easy recognition of doctors
they are a badge of office

against;
they act as a barrier between doctor and patient
they can act as a reservoir of infection if not changed frequently
surveys suggest patients do not like them

What problems do you think the widespread use of recreational drugs pose to doctors?

There are a number of issues relating to doctors, the first is the possibility of doctors themselves being exposed to recreational drugs and with access to drugs such as diamorphine (heroine) used for pain control there is a risk of addiction amongst doctors. With regard to patients recreational drugs pose a diagnostic problem if the user is not forthcoming about what they have used. There have been several high profile deaths from ecstasy use amongst teenagers, this usually presents as a coma secondary to water intoxication and can prove difficult to diagnose quickly without a good history. Extensive drug usage tends to lead to infections and malnutrition. IV drug users suffer the risk of hepatitis B, C and HIV infection from dirty needles. Tuberculosis is making a come back partly due to HIV making people more susceptible. Some

Female infertility treatment is expensive, has a very low success rate and is even less successful in smokers. To whom do you think it should be available?

Availability of infertility treatment varies between PCTs most decline it if a couple have a child. Many restrict it to one or two attempts, some agree to pay for the expensive drugs used only. It is unreasonable to restrict it to non-smokers as discussed earlier (GMC guidance). There is an argument as to whether infertility is a disease that should be treated on the NHS or a lifestyle choice that should be paid for by an individual. You might argue against a 'postcode lottery' and for a countrywide decision on such issues. There is talk in the papers, presumably leaked by government that non-essential treatments will need to be paid for by patients.

Can you give me an example of how you coped with a conflict with a colleague or friend; what strategy did you use and why?

This is all about how you manage difficult situations.
Here is some advice on conflict resolution if you are not so good at it!

Set the Scene
Make sure that people understand that the conflict may be a mutual problem, which may be best resolved through discussion and negotiation rather than aggression.

Emphasize the fact that you are presenting your perception of the problem. Use active listening skills to ensure you hear and understand other's positions and perceptions.

Restate
Paraphrase
Summarize
And make sure that when you talk, you're using an adult, assertive approach rather than a submissive or aggressive style.

Gather Information
Ask for the other person's viewpoint and confirm that you respect his or her opinion and need his or her cooperation to solve the problem. Try to understand his or her motivations and goals, and see how your actions may be affecting these.

Try to understand the conflict in objective terms: Is it disrupting team work? hampering decision-making? or so on. Be sure to focus on work issues and leave personalities out of the discussion.

Listen with empathy and see the conflict from the other person's point of view

Identify issues clearly and concisely
Use "I" statements, 'I feel we might be moving forward here'
Remain flexible
Clarify feelings

Agree the Problem
Often different underlying needs, interests and goals can cause people to perceive problems very differently. You'll need to agree the problems that you are trying to solve before you'll find a mutually acceptable solution.

Brainstorm Possible Solutions
If everyone is going to feel satisfied with the resolution, it will help if everyone has had fair input in generating solutions. Brainstorm possible solutions, and be open to all ideas, including ones you never considered before.

Negotiate a Solution

By this stage, the conflict may be resolved: Both sides may better understand the position of the other, and a mutually satisfactory solution may be clear to all.

There are three guiding principles here: Be Calm, Be Patient, Have Respect…

Have you ever been in a situation where you realise afterwards that what you said or did was wrong? What did you do about it? What should you have done?

It is crucial that doctors are able to say 'sorry' when they make a mistake. The vast majority of litigation cases are brought, not because a mistake has been made, they happen all the time. It is because there is a perceived cover up or a denial of blame or a lack of apology. This question is designed to look at attitude and it is important you are quick to explain and apologise and negotiate a resolution

Give us an example of something about which you used to hold strong opinions, but have had to change your mind. What made you change? What do you think now?

Tricky one and one you will wish you had planned an answer to. This is looking at how rigidly you hold beliefs and whether you can compromise. It might be a religious, cultural or racial belief.

What is your opinion on "Widening access to Medicine courses?"

Here it is probably a good idea to bang on about the importance of all sectors of society having access to medical courses if they have the intellect. The reason for this is the need for patients to be able to relate to their doctor and in a meritocracy people should be able to reach their potential without class barriers inhibiting them. Education is a major issue with colleges reducing their admission standards for state-school educated children which has led to Oxbridge laying a charge of dumming down which might lead to them seeking independent status. The argument for the policy is that public school pupils are given far more assistance in passing examinations and parental support.

What happens between the time a pharmacist invents a drug and a doctor prescribing it.

Once a drug is discovered it is tested in non-human models, either cell lines or animals. Once the safety and pharmacokinetics (the half life, likely dosage required) are established in animals the drug is tested in healthy volunteers (phase 1 trial). This establishes safety in a limited way and the possible human dose. If the drug passes these it enters phase 2 trials, in humans with the disease being treated, against either a placebo or the currently used drug or both. If this is completed phase

3 trials in large numbers of patients begin, these are hugely costly and confirm whether the drug works, safety and dose. If the drug passes this it is put before the panel that decides if it is to be licensed. Onc on the market, phase 4, reporting of adverse effects occurs.

What are the pros and cons of pharmaceutical representatives visiting doctors to promote their drugs?

The advantages are that they keep one up to date with new drug developments. You might argue that this can be done by reading and attending conferences but this may not be a simple option for some.

The disadvantages are that the information provided is carefully edited to give a good impression of the drug. Trials quoted are often small and insignificant, side effects may be minimised and benefits exaggerated. The influence that drug reps have over prescribing has led to significant changes in the rules under which pharma companies have to work. Expensive meals, trips away and gifts are now severely restricted.

Index

A

Aberdeen 13, 20
advantages and disadvanta 187
advantages and disadvantages of being in a team? 200
application process. 13

B

Barts and The London, QMUL 20, 34
Birmingham 20, 35, 102
blogs 74
BMAT 13, 14, 15, 16, 21, 24, 28, 30, 35, 108, 161, 162, 163, 164
Body language 76
Brighton and Sussex 13, 21, 103
Brighton and Sussex Medical School 103
Bristol 21, 31, 35, 39, 103, 104, 105, 106, 109, 175, 182

C

'choose and book' 199
Cambridge 14, 21, 22, 35, 37, 58, 107, 108, 125
Cardiff 13, 22, 32, 38, 110, 157
Choosing a medical school 6, 38
Cloning 259
cloning 193, 258
confidentiality 85, 164, 179, 193, 224, 229, 234, 247, 248, 249, 251, 252

D

difficult patient 256
drugs 267

Index

Dundee 22
Durham 13, 22, 111
duties of a doctor 224

E

East Anglia 13, 23, 111, 112
Edinburgh 13, 23, 32, 53, 58, 70, 107, 112, 113, 127, 129, 145, 156
Entry Examinations 13
Ethical Scenario 77, 112, 137
Ethical scenarios 192, 227
European working time directive 200
euthanasia 230

F

Foundation Year 243

G

GAMSAT 14, 16, 17, 37, 38
GAP year 51, 71
Glasgow 13, 23, 110
global warming 193, 258
GMC 212
Graduate Entry 6, 8, 16, 34, 36, 38

H

herceptin 198
Hull York Medical School 13, 24, 114, 115
human genome project 190

I

Imperial College 24, 232
infertility treatment 122, 177, 194, 268
Interview 74

K

Keele 13, 24, 33, 132, 134, 243
Kings College London 16, 25, 33, 36

L

Lancaster 25
leader or a team player 187, 201
Leeds 13, 25, 39
Leicester 13, 26, 36, 138
limitations or weakness 187
Liverpool 25, 26, 36, 43, 138

M

Manchester 13, 26, 27, 30, 33, 38, 39, 90, 138, 141, 142, 143, 145, 146
medical school interviews 90
MMC 189, 199
Modernising Medical Careers 212

N

Newcastle Upon Tyne 27
nonessential surgery 214
Nottingham 13, 27, 34, 37, 70, 125, 148, 149, 150, 151, 152, 153

O

Oxford 13, 14, 26, 28, 33, 37, 56, 154

P

'payment by results' 199
PBL 211
Peninsula 13, 17, 28, 154
Personal Statement 1, 2, 6, 8, 45, 137
pharmaceutical representatives 194
Positive behavioural indicators 185
practice based commissioning 199

Q

Queens University Belfast 28

S

screening 132, 139, 141, 176, 192, 193, 235, 239
Sheffield 14, 29, 34, 155, 156
Southampton 14, 29, 37, 45, 63, 156
St. Andrews 29
stress 53, 68, 72, 79, 94, 105, 123, 124, 129, 142, 143, 144, 147, 149, 153, 155, 165, 172, 181, 185, 187, 201, 202, 258
St George's 14, 17, 30, 38, 166

T

theories of justice 214
tobacco 232

U

UCAS form 6, 41, 42, 44, 86, 101, 105
UKCAT 13, 14, 16, 20, 21, 22, 23, 24, 25, 26, 27, 28, 29, 30, 32, 33, 34, 36, 37
University College London 30, 156

W

Why have you chosen to do medicine 187
work experience 36, 50, 52, 53, 54, 56, 61, 64, 66, 68, 70, 71, 72, 79, 90, 92, 93, 94, 95, 97, 98, 99, 100, 101, 104, 105, 106, 108, 110, 111, 112, 117, 123, 125, 127, 128, 129, 131, 136, 137, 138, 141, 144, 145, 146, 149, 151, 152, 153, 157, 158, 159, 160, 161, 162, 163, 164, 166, 167, 169, 172, 178, 179, 180, 181, 188, 196, 197, 202, 203, 204